KU-713-833

Lecture Notes
Elderly Care Medicine

Claire Nicholl
MB FRCP
Consultant Physician and Associate Lecturer

K. Jane Wilson
MB FRCP
Consultant Physician and Associate Lecturer

Stephen Webster
MA MD FRCP
Consultant Emeritus

All of:
Department of Medicine for the Elderly
Addenbrooke's Hospital
Cambridge, UK

Seventh Edition

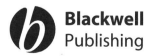

Blackwell
Publishing

© 2008 Claire Nicholl, K. Jane Wilson and Stephen Webster
Published by Blackwell Publishing
Blackwell Publishing, Inc., 350 Main Street, Malden, Massachusetts 02148-5020, USA
Blackwell Publishing Ltd, 9600 Garsington Road, Oxford OX4 2DQ, UK
Blackwell Publishing Asia Pty Ltd, 550 Swanston Street, Carlton, Victoria 3053, Australia

The right of the Author to be identified as the Author of this Work has been asserted in accordance with the Copyright, Designs and Patents Act 1988.

All rights reserved. No part of this publication may be reproduced, stored in a retrieval system, or transmitted, in any form or by any means, electronic, mechanical, photocopying, recording or otherwise, except as permitted by the UK Copyright, Designs and Patents Act 1988, without the prior permission of the publisher.

First published 1977
Second edition 1980
Third edition 1988
Fourth edition 1993
Fifth edition 1998
Sixth edition 2003
Seventh edition 2007

1   2008

Library of Congress Cataloging-in-Publication Data

Nicholl, Claire.
Lecture notes. Elderly care medicine / Claire Nicholl, K. Jane Wilson, Stephen Webster. -- 7th ed.
   p. ; cm.
Rev. ed. of: Lecture notes on geriatric medicine / Nicholas Coni ... [et al.]. 2003.
Includes bibliographical references and index.
ISBN 978-1-4051-5712-4 (alk. paper)
   1. Geriatrics--Outlines, syllabi, etc. I. Wilson, K. Jane (Kathryn Jane) II. Webster, Stephen.
   III. Lecture notes on geriatric medicine. IV. Title. V. Title: Elderly care medicine.
[DNLM: 1. Geriatrics. 2. Aged. WT 100 N595L 2007]

RC952.C583 2007
618.97--dc22
                                                                2007020965

ISBN: 978-1-4051-5712-4

A catalogue record for this title is available from the British Library

Set in Stone Serif 8/12 pts by Newgen Imaging Systems Pvt Ltd, Chennai, India
Printed and bound in Singapore by Utopia Press Pte Ltd

Commissioning Editor: Martin Sugden
Editorial Assistant: Robin Harries
Development Editor: Hayley Salter
Production Controller: Debbie Wyer

For further information on Blackwell Publishing, visit our website:
http://www.blackwellpublishing.com

Site	MIDDLESEX UNIVERSITY LIBRARY
WH	
Accession No.	07079664
Class No.	WT 100 NIC
Special Collection ✓	

The publisher's policy is to use permanent paper from mills that operate a sustainable forestry policy, and which has been manufactured from pulp processed using acid-free and elementary chlorine-free practices. Furthermore, the publisher ensures that the text paper and cover board used have met acceptable environmental accreditation standards.

Designations used by companies to distinguish their products are often claimed as trademarks. All brand names and product names used in this book are trade names, service marks, trademarks or registered trademarks of their respective owners. The Publisher is not associated with any product or vendor mentioned in this book.

Contents

Preface

Welcome to the seventh edition of this volume. In rewriting we have had to remove or correct very little – this is a reflection of our aim to only use evidence-based information. However, the continuing progress of medicine, in general, and geriatrics, in particular, has made it necessary to add some additional material. We have striven to keep the expansion to a minimum to ensure the book remains user-friendly.

It is now over 30 years since the first edition. During this time, we have attempted to guide an entire generation of doctors in the medical care of elderly patients. We now hope to influence the next generation in the forthcoming decades. During these 30 years, medicine and the specialty have developed considerably. Geriatric medicine has grown in stature, complexity and respectability to the extent that it is now the largest adult specialty in medical practice.

Many geriatricians have now developed special interests within the overall specialty. However, we must guard against repeating the mistakes of general medicine. We must never stray from our prime purpose of assisting, guiding and helping the most vulnerable of patients in old age. The giants of geriatric medicine described by Bernard Isaacs still cast their shadows over the end of life (see page 26) and we must not ignore them or neglect to combat them at the same time as extending to elderly patients as many as possible of the advances achieved in medicine since the first edition of this book. During these days when target-driven policies inflicted from above have a tendency to displace the genuinely important by the artificially urgent, it is essential that we remain true to our original aims and ideas.

We hope that contemporary doctors will find this book as useful as did their predecessors.

List of abbreviations

AA	Alcoholics Anonymous
ABGs	arterial blood gases
ACA	anterior cerebral artery
ACE	angiotensin-converting enzyme
ACEi	ACE inhibitor
AChE	acetylcholinesterase
ACS	acute coronary syndrome
ACTH	adrenocorticotrophic hormone
AD	Alzheimer's disease
ADL	activities of daily living
ADs	advance decisions/directives
AED	antiepileptic drug
AF	atrial fibrillation
AFB	acid-fast bacilli
AIDP	acute inflammatory demyelinating polyradiculoneuropathy
AMPA	α-amino-3-hydroxy-5-methylisoxa-zole-4-propionic acid receptor
AMT	Abbreviated Mental Test
ANS	autonomic nervous system
AP	antero-posteriorly
ARB	angiotensin receptor blocker
ARMD	Age-related macular degeneration
AV	atrioventricular
AVP	arginine vasopressin
Aβ	amyloid beta-peptide
BCC	basal-cell carcinoma
BMA	British Medical Association
BMI	body mass index
BMD	bone mineral density
BNF	British National Formulary
BP	blood pressure
BPH	benign prostatic hypertrophy
BPSD	behavioural and psychological symptoms
CADASIL	cerebral autosomal dominant arteriopathy with subcortical infarcts and leucoencephalopathy
CAPD	continuous ambulatory peritoneal dialysis
CBD	corticobasal degeneration
CCF	congestive cardiac failure
CCU	coronary care unit
CHARM	The Candesartan in Heart Failure Assessment of Reduction in Morbidity and Mortality
CIDP	chronic inflammatory demyelinating polyradiculoneuropathy
CK-MB	creatine kinase with muscle and brain subunits
CLL	chronic lymphocytic leukaemia
CNS	central nervous system
COHb	carboxyhaemoglobin
COPD	chronic obstructive pulmonary disease
COX-2	cyclo-oxygenase-2
CPN	Community Psychiatric Nurse
CPR	cardio-pulmonary resuscitation
CRP	C-reactive protein
CSF	cerebrospinal fluid
CVA	cerebrovascular accident
CVP	central venous pressure
CXR	chest X-ray
DC	direct current
DEXA	dual-energy X-ray absorptiometry
DGH	District General Hospital
DIC	disseminated intravascular coagulation
DIP	distal interphalangeal
DLB	dementia with Lewy bodies
DMARDs	disease-modifying anti-rheumatic drugs
DNR	do not resuscitate
DVLA	Driver and Vehicle Licensing Authority
DVT	deep vein thrombosis
ECG	electrocardiogram
ECT	electroconvulsive therapy
eGFR	estimated glomerular filtration rate
EMG	electromyogram
EOFAD	early-onset familial Alzheimer's disease

ERCP	endoscopic retrograde cholangiopancreatography
ESR	erythrocyte sedimentation rate
FBC	full blood count
FEV1	forced expiratory volume in 1 s
FSH	follicle stimulating hormone
FVC	forced vital capacity
GDNF	glial cell-line derived nerve growth factor
GDP	gross domestic product
GDS	Geriatric Depression Score
GFR	glomerular filteration rate
GI	gastrointestinal
GLP-1	glucagon-like peptide
GORD	gastro-oesophageal reflux disease
GP	general practitioner
GTN	glyceryl trinitrate
HOOF	Home Oxygen Order Form
HUT	head-up tilt
IHD	ischaemic heart disease
IBS	irritable bowel syndrome
IC	intermediate care
ICA	internal carotid artery
IMCA	independent mental capacity advocates
INR	international normalised ratio
ITU	intensive therapy unit
LacI	lacunar infarct
LH	luteinising hormone
LMN	lower-motor-neuron
LMWH	low-molecular-weight heparin
LOAD	late-onset Alzheimer's disease
LOC	loss of consciousness
LP	lumbar puncture
LPA	lasting power of attorney
LTOT	long-term oxygen therapy
LV	left ventricular
LVH	left ventricular hypertrophy
MCA	Mental Capacity Act
MCA	middle cerebral artery
MDS	myelodysplastic syndrome
MGUS	monoclonal gammopathy of unknown significance
MHA	Mental Health Act
MI	myocardial infarction
MMSE	Mini-Mental State Examination
MNA	Mini-Nutritional Assessment
MND	motor-neuron disease
MPTP	1-methyl-4-phenyl-1,2,3, 4-tetrahydropyridine
MRSA	methicillin-resistant Staphylococcus aureus
MS	multiple sclerosis
MSU	midstream urine
MTP	metatarso-phalangeal
NAFLD	non-alcoholic fatty liver disease
NBM	nil by mouth
NCS	nerve conduction studies
NCSE	non-convulsive status epilepticus
NG	nasogastric
NHS	National Health Service
NHS CC	NHS continuing care
NICE	National Institute for Health and Clinical Excellence
NMDA	N-methyl-d-aspartate
NOF	neck of femur
NSAID	non-steroidal anti-inflammatory drug
NSCLC	non-small-cell lung cancer
NSF OP	National Service Framework for Older People
NSTEMI	non-ST-elevation infarcts
OA	osteoarthritis
OGD	oesophago gastro duodenoscopy
PA	pernicious anaemia
PACI	partial anterior circulatory infarct
PBC	primary biliary cirrhosis
PBR	payment by result
PCR	polymerase chain reaction
PCT	primary care trust
PD	Parkinson's disease
PE	pulmonary embolism
PEG	percutaneous endoscopic gastrostomy
PICC	peripherally inserted central catheter
PIP	proximal interphalangeal joints
PMR	polymyalgia rheumatica
PoCI	posterior circulatory infarct
PPARγ	peroxisome-proliferator-activated receptor gamma
PPS	post-polio syndrome
PSA	prostate-specific antigen
PTCA	percutaneous transluminal coronary angioplasty
PTH	parathyroid hormone
PUVA	psoralen + UVA treatment

PVS	persistent vegetative state	TACI	total anterior circulatory infarct
QOF	quality and outcomes framework	TB	tuberculosis
RA	rheumatoid arthritis	TEDS	thromboembolic deterrant stockings
RAS	renal artery stenosis	TENS	transcutaneous electrical nerve
RCP	Royal College of Physicians		stimulation
RoSPA	Royal Society for the Prevention of	TFT	thyroid-function test
	Accidents	TIA	transient ischaemic attack
rt-PA	recombinant-tissue-type	TOE	transoesophageal echocardiography
	plasminogen	tPA	tissue plasminogen activator
SAH	subarachnoid haemorrhage	TSH	thyroid stimulating hormone
SCC	squamous-cell carcinoma	TURP	transurethral prostatectomy
SCLC	small-cell lung cancer	TVT	tension-free vaginal tape
SD	standard deviation	U & E	urea and electrolyte
SE	status epilepticus	UKPDS	United Kingdom Prospective Diabetes
SERM	selective estrogen modulator		Study
SLE	systemic lupus erythematosus	UMN	upper-motor-neuron
SN	substantia nigra	UTI	urinary-tract infection
SOL	space-occupying lesion	VEGF	vascular endothelial growth factor
SSRI	selective serotonin reuptake	VTE	venous thromboembolism
	inhibitor	WBC	white blood cell
STEMI	ST-elevation myocardial infarcts	YAG	Yittrium Aluminium Garnet

Chapter 1

The world grows old

Introduction

If the 20th century was the period when the Western world turned grey, it is to be hoped that the 21st century will be the time when it wakes up to the new situation and begins to make appropriate plans for services. There is some evidence that this is occurring. The increasing presence of elderly people is now recognized in plays, films, soap operas and comedy series.

The common afflictions of old age are now well recognized, not as a cause for shame and disgrace, but as serious diseases. Examples include the public information about the dementia of ex-President Reagan of the USA and a dramatization of the same disease as it affected the famous philosopher and novelist Iris Murdoch. Middle-aged, middle-class articulate 'children' such as Michael Ignatief, Linda Grant and Margaret Mason have written in detail about the dementing process as it affected their parents, themselves and their families. John Mortimer has described the problems associated with visual impairment in his elderly father and he now writes amusingly about his own infirmities of old age.

The Human Rights Act 1998 (2000) has the potential to offer protection to vulnerable elderly people, especially Articles 2, 3, 8, 10 and 14 (see the following box). This Act applies to all public bodies, i.e. the NHS and Local Authority Social Service Departments.

Human rights act 1998

Article 2 Right to life.
Article 3 Prohibition of torture and inhuman and degrading treatment.
Article 8 Right to respect for private and family life and home.
Article 10 Freedom of expression and right to information.
Article 14 Right not to be discriminated against.

Population trends

There are marked differences between the developed and developing countries, e.g. France took 115 years (1865–1980) to double the proportion of elderly people (7–14%) whereas China's proportion will double between 2000 and 2027. The prime reason for the worldwide increase in the proportion of elderly subjects is the combined effect of declining child mortality and a falling birth rate. Consequences and solutions will depend on the levels of economic and educational development within individual countries. By 2030 most countries will have a similar age structure. See Table 1.1 for the predicted elderly population of 2025.

Developed countries

• There has been a dramatic rise in the elderly throughout the past 100 years, but this is now slowing down (Figure 1.1).

1

Table 1.1 Predicted elderly population (over 65 years in thousands) in 2025.

China	198,343
India	107,713
Indonesia	24,816
Brazil	21,945
Mexico	12,829
UK	12,912
Nigeria	9,115

- However, the 'old old', i.e. those greater than 75 years of age, are still increasing rapidly. In the UK the over-85s will continue to double every 30 years (1961, 300,000; 1991, 800,000; 2021, 1,500,000).
- A sophisticated medical service is established.
- Specialist services are available for the elderly.
- The rising expectations of the elderly, their supports and carers will result in rising costs.
- Population trends in the UK alone demand a 1% increase in health funding in addition to inflation and costs due to technological development.
- Ethical dilemmas will be more pressing, e.g. the prolongation of death by technological intervention or medicated survival of the young chronically sick and acutely ill, frail, elderly patients.

- Financial consequences of decisions must be calculated and proper provisions must be made to support the choice made. An elderly person costs the health services nine times as much as a young person.
- A century ago, i.e. in 1900, more children under 1 year of age died each year than people under the age of 65 now die each year – see Table 1.2 showing changes in the death rate over time.
- By 2015, in the UK, it is predicted that people over the age of 65 will begin to outnumber those under 16 years of age.
- The Commission on Global Ageing warns of the risk of 'ageing recessions' due to a fall in the size of workforce numbers (labour shortages) plus increased service demands (caring services). The peak risk is expected in 2010, but Japan has already been affected.
- Increasing anxiety exists concerning future poverty in old age, due to shrinkage in state benefits, reluctance of 'the young' to invest in pension schemes and the unreliability of financial services in regard to pension provision.
- Medical training continues to concentrate on increasing super-/sub-specialization, thus leading to practitioners being unable to cope with complex

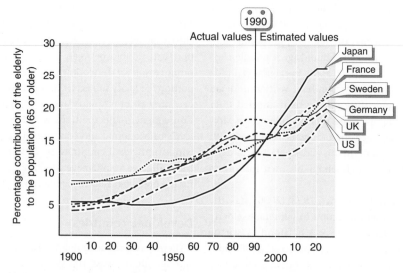

Figure 1.1 Elderly as percentage of population (65 or older).

Table 1.2 UK mortality rates for young and old.

1919	12% of deaths in first year of life; 65% of deaths before the age of 65 years
2002	<1% of deaths in first year of life; 19% of deaths before the age of 65 years

Note: Death, formerly common in infancy and usual before 65 years, is now rare in infancy and unusual before 65 years.

aetiologies (sociological, psychological and medical) and multi-pathology (co-morbidity), and the atypical presentations common in elderly patients, i.e. a mismatch between aspirations of young medics and the needs of their elderly patients.

• Community care is quite rightly individually based and very varied. Comparisons between countries is therefore very difficult because of variations in taxation policy, population density and political climate. It is, however, easier to make comparisons with regard to institutional care, usually in residential or nursing homes. Even here there are wide variations from the UK, with 4% of the persons over 65 years of age in care homes compared with the USA, at almost 6%, and the Netherlands, at almost 11%.

• The historical development of the patterns of care are similar. In all societies, there has always been a heavy reliance on self-sufficiency and family care. In these circumstances, the healthy old and the wealthy old have always faired the best. For the more disadvantaged, there has always been a need to rely on support from non-family members.

• In the 'Old World', this non-family support was originally provided by the church or by occupationally related charities or guilds. In England, the state began to become more prominent in the 17th century with the first Poor Law Act, which provided workhouse care and 'outdoor relief' (through community support, usually financial). This continued until the end of the 19th century. The 20th century saw the beginning of the welfare state – gradually growing in the first half of the century and reaching a peak at mid-century and then declining towards the end of the 1980s. At the time of decline, the general move was away from the provision of services by the state to the regulation of provision of services supplied by other organizations. This regulation has gradually been devolved and often diluted with the central control gradually lost or weakened. This trend has been most marked in the USA, but is now apparent in Australasia and the UK.

• In the USA, 67% of nursing homes are run by profit-making organizations (increasingly large multinational companies). In 1999, one of the largest companies also had large numbers of beds in Europe and Australia. However, the for-profit companies have a worse record for staffing levels (20% less than non-profit-making institutions) and skill mix, and a higher incidence of violations of standards. The regulatory arrangements are clearly failing to improve or even maintain standards. Public control appears to have been lost and for every dollar spent in the for-profit area, less than 26 cents is spent on care.

• In Australia, the proportion of for-profit nursing home beds was historically about 27%, but had risen to 55% by the year 2000. Between 1996 and 2000, the cost of public funding of private nursing homes rose from A$2.5 to A$3.9 billion. The cost of the regulatory system has doubled, but it appears to be weakening as unannounced inspections ceased, reports of inspections became more difficult to obtain and available sanctions were rarely used.

Developing countries

• These countries currently have 50% of the world's elderly population – which will rise to 75% by the year 2020.

• These countries are about to experience a massive and rapid distortion of previous population patterns, the rate of increase in the elderly population will be up to 15 times that of the UK (e.g. in Colombia, the Philippines and Thailand).

• The rising number of elderly people will coincide with falling birth rate, as contraceptive policies become effective.

• Their health services are often primitive, patchy and inappropriate to needs.

• There are many other pressing financial demands for expansion, e.g. education, housing and development of infrastructure.

- Economic dependence on developed countries is restrictive.
- Political instability is common.
- Social structure is likely to be rapidly altered, e.g. by population migration and reduced infant mortality.
- Potentially preventable disabilities acquired in youth will complicate old age.
- The poor will be unable to acquire sufficient wealth to provide for themselves in old age; therefore, the total burden will either fall on the state or will be neglected.
- European studies show that the survival of babies with low birth-weight and reduced growth in the first year leads to poor adult health – especially regarding BP and blood sugar control. This is likely to have significant consequences in India and Southeast Asia in the future.
- Globalization via the World Trade Organization will attempt to maintain high drug costs and introduce insurance schemes that will cherry-pick the affluent or well-off and leave the disadvantaged to the struggling public services. There is also likely to be encouragement of inappropriate 'high-tech' procedures. World trade also tends to encourage development of bad health habits; e.g. smoking tobacco, excess use of alcohol and the recreational use of drugs.
- Population patterns at risk of distortion by epidemics, e.g. HIV/AIDS.
- It is a false assumption that elderly people in undeveloped countries are not a problem because they are so few. They do exist and their life expectancy at 65 years is very similar in both developed and undeveloped countries (see Table 1.3).
- Doctors and nurses training in the undeveloped countries need expertise in elderly care because of the changing demography of their own countries and the tendency for them to be 'poached' by

Population of UK			
	1971	1996	2061
<16 years old	25%	21%	17%
>65 years old	13%	16%	24%

In 2015, the population aged <16 years will equal the population aged >65 years.

Population of India
Year 2000 7% over 60 years of age.
Year 2025 12% over 60 years of age.

developed countries where they may find themselves confronted by very elderly patients for the first time.

Ageing in India

The descriptions of facilities for 'care' in this book (as opposed to 'cure') of elderly people will be representative of the Western world, especially of the UK. This is because national variation is great and space is limited. With regard to the less developed countries, information is often very limited and sometimes unreliable. These restrictions apply to information about India, but at least statistics are being collected. To illustrate some of the differences between the East and the West, we have included information from the WHO publication *Ageing in India*, published in 1999. Life expectancy at the age of 60 in India has increased for both men and women between 1961 and 2001 by 3–4 years, and is now 15.2 years for men and 16.4 years for women. The box below shows commonest diseases and disabilities in the elderly population in India. It should be noted that, as is the case worldwide, cardiovascular disease takes pole position. Some 60–75% of elderly people in India are economically dependent, usually on their families. However, the extended family is disappearing and the social status of elderly people is being eroded. Since 1992, an old age pension has been available for those with no means of support at a level of approximately US$1.00 per month. Services for elderly

Table 1.3 Life expectancy at 65 years.

	Developed countries (Years)	Undeveloped countries (Years)
Women	19	15
Men	16	12

Disease and disability in the over 60s in India

- Cardiovascular disease commonest cause of death in old age.
- 11 million elderly blind people – 80% due to cataract.
- 60% have hearing impairment.
- 9 million have hypertension.
- 5 million have diabetes.
- 0.35 million have cancer.
- 4 million have mental health problems.

Source: WHO report, *Ageing in India*, 1999.

---

people are very few and far between. In 1997, there was reported to be only 354 old people's homes, usually organized by charities.

Ageing in Africa

Ageing in Africa is different to that in other areas. It provides an example of how the unexpected can undermine projections. The effects of AIDS and war are seriously distorting the age patterns of this continent.

Africa is ageing more rapidly than any other region (four times the rate of Europe). In spite of this, life expectancy is falling! The latter is due to 19–25% of the adult population being HIV-positive plus a two-fold increase in child mortality. The surviving elderly grandmothers (head of family in 43% of Zimbabwian families with AIDS orphans) are increasingly left behind in rural areas to care for HIV/AIDS infected children and grandchildren. Meanwhile, fit middle-generation members migrate to the cities. The elderly in Africa are not themselves immune to HIV infection, but exact incidence is unknown. When contracted by an older person, the illness tends to run a more rapidly progressive decline. In addition, they are likely to find themselves without any informal carers or supporters.

The UN reports indicate that half of the teenagers in Africa will die from AIDS. In Botswana about two-thirds of 15 year olds will die before reaching the age of 50.

A WHO Report of 2001 calculated that the annual worldwide rate of war casualties is about one-third of a million, and that over half of these (54%) will occur in Africa and that the majority of victims will be between 15 and 45 years of age.

Ageing in Brazil

Here disability rises with increasing age as elsewhere. The prevalence of the difficulty in walking and performance of personal care is similar to that found in the UK (especially in men). However, those with less education and wealth were almost twice as likely to suffer from disability compared with their peers. Urban dwellers were also more disabled than those in rural areas.

Ageing in Malaysia

This region is not excluded from the worldwide increase in the elderly population (about 2.5% per annum in those over 65 years of age who now total about 1 million or 4.5% of the total population). The current health services are a mixture of private and Government provision based on a network of 13 state general hospitals with Kuala Lumpur General Hospital acting as the tertiary referral centre but with support from the University Teaching Hospitals.

Most general practitioners work on a fee-based system and function as private practitioners. The current emphasis is on acute care with little rehabilitation provision. However, 44% of the patients attending the University Hospital family practice clinic are aged over 60 years. Nationally, there are only nine geriatricans (2004) and most are based in the capital city and concentrate on research and teaching.

A strong nursing service exists but appears reluctant to become involved in elderly care. Most 'care' is provided by family members, but it is becoming increasingly acceptable to place elders within a nursing home after an acute episode of illness.

Global warming

The Kyoto protocol came into force in 2005. It is predicated that if greenhouse gas emissions are not reduced the health burdens of climate change are likely to double by 2020 (*CMAJ* 2005, **172**, 501–2). Elderly people will not be excluded from these changes. In fact, the experience from France in the 2-week summer heat-wave of 2003 indicates that elderly people are the most vulnerable group. Most deaths occur in people over 70 and within the first few days of a heat-wave. Preventative measures are therefore needed and should be taken when a heat-wave is forecast. The death rate in France showed an estimated excess death rate in August 2003 of 13,600 with perhaps 5000 deaths being caused by the excessive heat. These deaths were not through hyperthermia but due to unbearable stress on already strained homeostatic cardiac and respiratory systems.

There is also a fear that diarrhoeal diseases may become more frequent with higher environmental temperatures. The vulnerability of frail elderly people with their inability to withstand severe and prolonged diarrhoea is well established.

It has been suggested that it will be through the mechanism of extreme climatic events rather than a steady change (2–3°C temperature rise by 2100) which will cause the major stress on the health of vulnerable populations. It should be noted that HelpAge International reported in the 2004 tsunami in Asia that some of the major losses were amongst the elderly section of the population. About 92,000 people over the age of 60 were displaced. In addition, these elderly people appeared to become almost invisible when aid was provided. They were often pushed aside by younger and fitter survivors during the chaotic distribution of relief.

Similar experiences were reported from the Orissa cyclone of 1999 and the Gujarat earthquake of 2001. Significant deficiencies also related to the provision of treatment for patients with chronic conditions. Monetary supplements, special diets and psychological support were also lacking, especially for elderly people.

Global poverty

Although the West complains about the detrimental effects of diseases of affluence, the situation on a global scale seems quite different (see Table 1.4). However, affluence in the UK appears to have enhanced the life expectancy difference between the highest and lowest social classes between 1972 and 1999 (see Table 1.6). Comparing continents, there appears to be an association between wealth (gross domestic product – GDP) and life expectancy at birth. Africa being the poorest and with the worst life expectancy. The latter has been reduced by the ravages of AIDS but the global differences persist when the contribution of AIDS is removed (see Table 1.4).

Inter generational strife

This is a potential problem which all must strive to avoid in both developed and under-developed countries. Strains and conflict could arise due to the falling dependency ratio (i.e. fewer working people to support those in need of care). There is the prospect of poverty in old age for the current young due to increased life expectancy but a decline in provision for

Table 1.4 Relationship between wealth and life expectancy at birth in various geographical areas.

		Life expectancy at birth	
	GDP in 2000	With AIDS	Without AIDS
Africa	2	50.6	56.9
Asia	4	67.7	68.3
Latin America and Caribbean	6	71.8	72.3
Oceania	21	74.6	74.6
Europe	14	74.3	74.6
North America	27	77.6	77.9

Table 1.5 Percentages of older people able to perform (ADL) independently at different ages.

	Age	1976 (%)	1991 (%)
Men	75–79	75	90
	85+	57	80
Women	75–79	67	90
	85+	52	80

Table 1.6 Widening gap in life expectancy at 65 in the UK, 1972–1999 (in days).

Social class	1972	1999	Increase
I	5200	6388	1188
V	4300	4891	591

pension payments (compared with current retirees). There is also an increased expectation of those growing old in the next two decades, e.g. aspiring early retirement with decreased disability levels (see Table 1.5) but still expecting enhanced care services.

Social aspects of ageing

Old age is unfortunately often a time of loss. The potential losses are very varied but are often inter-related, and those that accompany old age are of:
• Health due to increasing pathology.
• Wealth due to termination of employment.
• Companionship following bereavement.
• Independence due to acquired disabilities.
• Homoeostasis due to impairments to autonomic nervous system and renal function.
• Status following retirement and loss of independence.

The above changes and losses may expose the elderly person to the following consequences:
• Unhappiness, grief, depression, suicide (see Chapters 4 and 16).
• Increased incidence of illness.
• Increased risk of accident.
• Poverty.
• Dependence and abuse.
• Malnutrition and subnutrition.
• Hypothermia (see Chapter 12).

Loss of wealth

Income falls on giving up paid employment. Pensions are not normally equivalent to wages and the average pension is approximately 50% of the average working wage for a couple. Disabilities themselves may result in additional costs, e.g. for help, aids and adaptations.

The elderly spend a much higher percentage of their total expenditure on essentials, e.g. heating, food and housing, and there is little opportunity to economize. In the UK, the safety net provided by the social security system is complex and difficult and this alone acts as a deterrent to taking up available benefits. Occupational pensions and investment income are increasing in importance, but in the UK 50% of pensioners receive 75% of their income from the state pension.

Retirement

Retirement is a mixed blessing: 20% of workers fear retirement but 50% look forward to it. Retirement is a potential period of loss – of income, status, companionship and self-confidence.

To counteract the disadvantages, there are the following positive aspects of retirement:
• It may occupy one-third of life.
• Many remain fit and healthy for most of this time.
• It is an opportunity to redesign lifestyle and to promote good health.
• Time is available for new or renewed interests, activities and relationships.

But retirement may bring social problems of its own and it is a time when some difficult decisions will have to be made. Dilemmas encountered may include the following:
• Becoming a carer, e.g. of parents or grandchildren early in retirement or of spouse or siblings later on.
• Where to live – it is probably best to stay put where comfortable and well known. If a move is contemplated, earlier is better than later, as the retiree is likely to be fitter and one of a pair.
• What sort of accommodation? Somewhere where independence is possible, even in spite of acquired disabilities.

• Driving – may need to be given up at some stage, so beware of geographical isolation (see Chapters 5 and 16).

• Sex – it is 'allowed' even in very old age so long as it gives pleasure to both partners (see Chapter 13).

• Boredom affects 10% of the retired – another 20% (although not bored) would prefer still to be working. The poor, the disabled, the poorly educated and the isolated are most likely to be dissatisfied with retirement.

• The economic consequences of an expanding population of retired persons dependent on pensions are causing considerable worldwide concern within the developed world. As a consequence, the retirement age may well be gradually increased to 70+ years. In addition, there will also be a need to review the nature of paid employment in later years with consideration of plans to make partial or gradual retirement easier without loss of status, pay or pension rights. Preparation for retirement is vital.

• The increasing frailty and unpredictability of the global financial markets also pose threats to pension provision. The pension aspirations of many current workers may not be met and may be considered a potential threat to world finance.

Recommended physical activity in retirement

• Regular moderate intensity activity for 30 min on most days.
• Short bursts of exertion may have a cumulative effect.
• Start slow and gradually build up intensity and duration.
• If an activity is not provoking symptoms, it is unlikely to be doing harm.
• Generally benefits of activity outweigh risks.
• When activity requires special equipment or clothing, make sure it is appropriate and in good condition.

Some myths of ageing

• *It is a new problem*. No – there have always been elderly people, there are now just more of them.

In the past, most people were denied the opportunity of old age by dying young. Now, most babies born in the developed countries can expect to survive into their 80s.

• *All elderly people are decrepit and senile*. No – most live independent lives and mainly in their own homes (96% in the UK).

• *The chronic conditions of old age are untreatable*. No – medical treatment for all ages concerns itself primarily with the management of chronic conditions. The courses of disease can be slowed or modified – e.g. Parkinson's disease or senile dementia of the Alzheimer type – and symptoms can be alleviated – e.g. pain, breathlessness and in deficiency diseases (pernicious anaemia, osteomalacia and myxoedema) normal function can be restored.

• *Natural decline cannot be prevented*. No – regular physical activity in old age can rejuvenate and physical capacity can be improved by 10–15 years. Also, the adoption of a 'healthy lifestyle' in middle age (no smoking, avoidance of obesity and taking regular exercise) can delay the onset and decrease the eventual severity and duration of disability towards the end of life.

• *Treating elderly patients is a waste of money*. No – not to treat is not only inhumane (see Human Rights Act 1998) but often expensive, and neglected problems may lead to longer-term, higher expenditure (i.e. 'care' can be more expensive than 'cure').

• *Care of the elderly is bankrupting the NHS*. No – it is true that elderly people account for more costs within the NHS than the young (except for the management of children). However, most people make few demands on the NHS until the 15 years prior to their death. Costs for this terminal period are similar if death occurs at any age, i.e. 40, 50, 60 years, and so on. In fact, death in very old age may be gentle and not incur the high cost of unrealistic heroics.

• *All elderly people are depressed and lonely, and are better off dead*. No – the majority of elderly people are not depressed. In fact, well-being and contentment may feature in later life more than during the ambitious and frustrated productive years. Although the general population thinks that 90% of elderly people are lonely, only 10% of the elderly consider themselves to be so.

• *The elderly are of no use.* No – they are a valuable resource with experience and, sometimes, wisdom. The majority of carers are elderly and these include grandparents assisting in the rearing of their grandchildren because of absent or working parents. The old are the backbone of the voluntary services.

• *Old patients have a limited future and poor prognosis.* No – life expectancy at 65 years is in excess of 15 years. Survival for 5 years after many surgical and oncological treatments is recorded as a success.

Chapter 2

Health and social care for elderly people in the UK

How many older people are there?

The UK population topped 60 million for the first time in 2005. As well as increasing, the population is ageing, with the biggest percentage changes at extreme old age. The 2001 census was the first where the number of pensioners was greater than the number of children. In 2004, pensioners were estimated to make up 18.4% of the population. Different sources give figures for different age bands and areas, i.e. UK/Great Britain/England and Wales and after the census year (2001), most figures are estimates so you will find different numbers quoted. However, all agree that the proportion of the population aged 75+ and 85+ is increasing markedly and in line with this, the most dramatic change is seen in centenarians.

What is your life expectancy when you are old?

Life expectancy at extreme old age has always been longer than people think; a woman born in 1850 could expect another 4 years if she reached 80; for a women born in 1950 this is estimated to be 8.5 years. This is important for clinical management – an 80-year-old newly diagnosed diabetic will have time to develop complications! Currently, in the UK, a man of 65 can expect another 16.8 years of life and a woman, another 19.6 years. Unfortunately the figures for healthy life expectancy are not keeping pace, so although we are living longer, more of that time is not spent in a state of good or fairly good health, especially for women.

What are the characteristics of the older population?

Gender In the population aged 65+ (16% in 2006), women outnumber men because of their longer life expectancy and the death of young men in World War II. In 2003, there were 40 men per 100 women aged 85+, for 2031 the estimate is 65 per 100.

Ethnicity There is less ethnic mix than in the general population. Whereas, 12% people under 16 are

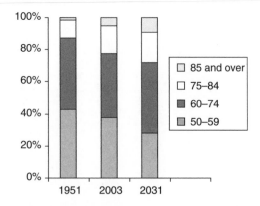

Figure 2.1 Percentage composition of the population aged 50+ in the UK, estimated for 2031, showing that within this group the population is ageing.

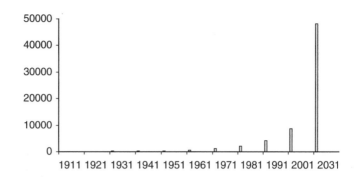

Figure 2.2 Numbers of centenarians between 1911 and 2031 (predicted) England and Wales.

from an ethnic minority group, this is 2.5% at 65+ and only 1% at 85+. However, 10% of Black Caribbean and 7% of Indian people were over 65 years in 2001.

Geographic variation Older people migrate from towns to the country and seaside so the distribution of people above state pension age (currently women of 60+ and men of 65+) is uneven. London is a young city. Three local authorities have more than 30% pensioners, the current leader being Christchurch in Dorset where a third of the population are pensioners.

Health status In the General Household Survey (2003), 60% of the sample aged 65–74 said they had a 'longstanding illness', which was felt to be 'limiting' in 37%. Aged 75+, the figures were 64% and 44%, respectively.

Sixty-six per cent of people registered blind are 75+ (2006).

Living companions In 2003, in Great Britain, 34% women and 19% men aged 65–74 lived alone

Table 2.1 Percentage of people in different age groups who live alone in Great Britain (General Household Survey, Office of National Statistics in Social Trends 36, 2006).

	% Men		% Women	
	1986–1987	2004–2005	1986–1987	2004–2005
75 and over	24	28	61	59
65–74	17	17	38	33
45–64	8	17	13	16
25–44	7	16	4	9
16–24	4	5	3	4

(Table 2.1). Aged 75+ this rose to 60% and 29%. White people are more likely to live alone than those from ethnic minority groups. One-third of pensioners live alone; half of them live with their spouses and only one-fifth live with children or siblings or friends. The multiple generation (extended family) is rare in the UK and probably has always been so.

Where do elderly people live?

The vast majority (95.5%) of people over 65 in the UK live in their own home (including sheltered flats). This is termed living in 'the community', in contrast with institutional care, although care homes should be part of the local community too! Owner-occupiers account for about 60%. A high percentage of elderly people (compared with the young) are in rented accommodation – about one-third in council property and half as many in the private sector. Results from the English House Condition Survey (2004) show that housing is steadily improving although 33.3% of people aged 75+ still live in a 'non-decent' home (versus 28.4% all households) and this age group are more likely to be in an energy-inefficient home (11.9% versus 8.4%), or a home in serious disrepair (11.2% versus 10.0%). Of the population over 65 years, 8% live in sheltered housing (Figure 2.3).

Sheltered housing

The usual pattern is a group of small flats (typically one bed, living room, kitchenette, bathroom and toilet) around communal facilities for meals or

11

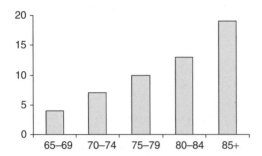

Figure 2.3 The marked effect of age on the percentage of people living in sheltered housing in Great Britain in 2001.

social activity, so residents have their own front door. Sheltered flats are provided by the local authority, housing associations and increasingly the private sector. There is a warden who may work office hours only. There is often a buzzer system so residents can summon help. Residents are usually able to wash, dress, transfer and mobilize independently (including wheelchair users) and prepare their own food. As residents are in their own home, they may have the usual services. Traditional sheltered accommodation is of most benefit to those with physical disability and very unsuitable housing. However, many schemes are being set up with staff on site round the clock to provide 'extra care' (for washing, dressing, meals, etc.). This enables much frailer residents to remain at home. There were around 20,000 places in 2005. Purpose-built developments may include components of 'assistive technology'.

Institutional care

Only 4.5% of people over 65 live in institutions, but this rate rises rapidly with increasing age to 12% aged over 75 years and 20% over 85 years. The rate in the UK is higher than in many continental European countries.

Institutionalization occurs when the person can no longer be supported at home *within the resources available* because of:

- Severe physical disabilities.
- Immobility without help.
- Severe mental disability as constant supervision is needed.

- Unpredictable and frequent care needs.

This point is reached sooner if the person has a passive personality and there is non-existent support or even hostility to the person remaining at home.

Complications of institutionalization include:

- Depersonalization.
- Marked restriction of choices.
- Accelerated dependence.

NB: All of these can be minimized by persistent effort by staff, visitors and sometimes the residents.

What types of institutions are there?

Long stay hospital

These have almost disappeared but they have left a difficult legacy in terms of who pays for care of this frailest group of old people. Successive governments struggle with the National Health Service (NHS) being 'free at the point of delivery', whereas care provided by social services has usually been means-tested. Twenty years ago, many elderly people spent their last months in a geriatric long stay hospital. This care had its limitations, but was free to the patient. With ever more exciting ways for the NHS to spend its budget, in some areas long stay hospitals were shut so patients were placed in nursing homes, transferring some of the costs to the individuals. Geographical variation in the availability of long-stay NHS beds resulted in inequity.

To try to restore equity, criteria were introduced to determine whether an individual was entitled to 'NHS Continuing Care' (NHS CC) for the remainder of their days. The term NHS CC is a specific piece of jargon, which relates to how care is paid for, not where it is provided. To fulfil the criteria, an individual is usually bed bound with multiple problems needing regular skilled nursing, e.g. for pressure sores or tube feeding and a very short prognosis. Decisions about eligibility are usually made by a local health and social care panel, so geographical variation persists. There is a right of appeal. This is used quite often, as if you have to pay for a nursing home, you may have to sell your house rather than leaving it to your family. If the patient is granted NHS CC, the actual care can be provided at home, in a nursing home or, occasionally, a hospital. The only country to take a fairer view is Scotland where the 'personal care' element is not separated from nursing care and is not means-tested. Many health professionals do not understand the specific use of the term NHS CC, and patients may be referred 'for assessment of continuing care' when advice is wanted about 'ongoing' care, i.e. might the person benefit from intermediate care or is placement appropriate?

Nursing homes

Most residents on entry are now over 80 years of age and suffer from multiple disabilities (both physical and mental) and need 'hotel services', i.e. help with personal hygiene and nursing care. Medical cover is provided by the resident's own general practitioner (GP). The move often results in the person having to change GP at a very vulnerable time. A registered nurse must be on duty 24 h a day. On admission, the person is usually chair or bed bound. The average weekly fee for a private nursing home bed is £455 (2003).

Residential homes

Residents need hotel services and help with personal hygiene and also have their own GP. Most of the staff are care assistants. On admission, a new client would usually be able to move from bed to chair with assistance and walk, perhaps, with help to the communal dining and sitting areas. Nursing care, if needed for a short period, is usually provided by a district nurse. The average weekly fee for a private care home bed is £329 (2003).

Residential homes and nursing homes are now all regulated by one authority, but the beds are registered for a specific client group. If a residential home resident becomes ill he or she may be admitted to hospital. The home can refuse to take the resident back 'as they can no longer meet their needs' and the unfortunate individual has to move again from the residential home to a nursing home. This causes much frustration as in this situation, the resident may have been declining for some time in the residential home; the wait for nursing home care increases length of stay and the

individual stuck in hospital may deteriorate further or even die from nosocomial infection. This situation is improved if the home has both nursing home and residential home beds. There is a lot of variation in the flexibility of both different homes and local authorities.

Specialist care home beds for elderly people with dementia

It is relatively easy to maintain a physically disabled but cognitively intact person at home – if problems arise between care visits they can summon help. While extra care sheltered flats with assistive technology (see above) can provide a good care setting, the commonest reason for people to need 24-h care is dementia on top of physical problems. Therefore, most nursing homes and residential homes will cope with a degree of dementia. However, if dementia is the main problem, in the form of wandering or disruptive behaviour, a specialist DeE (Dementia, elderly) residential home or nursing home will be needed.

Who provides institutional care?

Nursing home care is mainly provided by the private sector. There are a few NHS nursing homes. Residential home care was traditionally provided by local authorities, but is now also provided mainly by the private sector. There is some voluntary sector provision. It is a difficult market – the initial rapid increase in private beds has been followed by contraction. As more people are supported at home, patients entering institutional care are frailer and the costs outstrip the available funding. The major trends in bed provision are shown in Figure 2.4.

How is institutional care paid for?

In England and Wales, if an older person has enough savings, they can enter a private or voluntary sector home of their choice if they meet its admission criteria. If they need state financial support, they must first be assessed as needing institutional care and whether they need residential home or nursing home care (Figure 2.5). Then their

No. of places

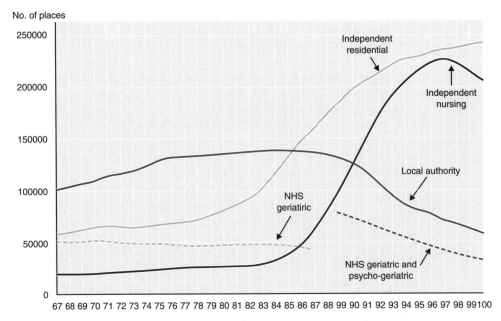

Figure 2.4 Long-term trends in the long-term care sector (adapted from Laing & Buisson, with permission).

financial situation is assessed. The individual has to contribute to the cost, ranging from forfeiting their allowances to paying the full amount for residential care if they have >£21,000 capital (2006). Residents must be left with a weekly personal allowance of £19.60. Owner-occupiers often have to sell to finance care unless a dependent relative continues to live in the house or insurance arrangements have been made. In a nursing home, the 'board and lodging' and 'personal care' components are means-tested but the state contributes to the 'registered nursing care contribution' at one of three levels depending on an assessment of

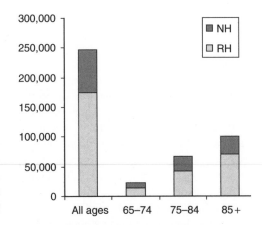

Figure 2.5 Council-supported residents in permanent residential and nursing care in England 2005.

nursing need. In a locality, the commissioners (social services/primary care trust – PCT) have a benchmark price for a nursing bed and a residential bed and a list of 'approved homes'. They may block purchase beds in a home. Approval is designed to improve standards but reduces choice, as does block-booking. Homes may be able to charge more in the private market so a social

---

Challenges for the UK care sector

1 Increasing numbers of old (i.e. >85 years).
2 Increasing frailty of residents – especially dementia with behavioural problems.
3 Staff recruitment and retention problems.
4 Financial consequences of increasing staff numbers, training and pay.
5 Rising public expectations.
6 Demands of recent legislation regarding space.
7 Inadequate benchmark funds.

services client can only get the bed if they or their family 'top-up' to pay the gap between the benchmark price and the price the home wishes to charge.

The number of council-supported residents fell by 3% from March 2005 to 2006. Of the supported residents, 61% were in independent residential care homes, 28% in independent nursing homes, and only 10% in council-staffed homes. Seventy-eight per cent of all supported residents were aged 65 or more.

How is care for older people organized?

Traditionally, health care was the responsibility of the NHS and social care of the social services department of the local authority; over the decades, the government departments responsible have been aggregated and disaggregated. All agencies providing services have a responsibility to older people – law and order, town planning, housing, transport, even education all impact on the quality of life and opportunities for older people.

Health care for older people

The organization of the NHS

This is immensely complex and is always being reorganized. In outline, England and Wales is divided into ten *Strategic Health Authorities*. Each of these contains around 15 *Primary Care Trusts* (PCTs) – in total 152. PCTs are tasked with assessing local need and *commissioning* care for their local population. This means buying care, according to contracts that specify the type, volume and quality aspects for different clinical problems, e.g. emergency admissions or elective cataract surgery. Many PCTs provided services themselves, but are now encouraged to separate these services from their 'main business' of commissioning. PCTs have to work with their councils on a local delivery plan to try to ensure that services are 'joined up'.

The NHS services to be commissioned include primary care (provided by GPs and their teams), a range of other community services, e.g. community hospitals, specialist nurses, secondary care

(traditionally provided in the DGH – District General Hospital) and tertiary care (specialist hospital care in regional or national centres, usually teaching hospitals). To complicate things, groups of GP practices (which are of course providing primary care) can be given the funding to commission the other care their patients need – this is called *Practice-based Commissioning*. GPs provide primary care for those with psychiatric problems but community, secondary and the rare tertiary mental health services are run by separate organizations.

The NHS hospitals are encouraged to gain more independence from government by becoming Foundation NHS Trusts. Once, a hospital had a budget to treat its local population. Payment for work done is now much more specific as hospitals move to *Payment by Results* (PBRs) – really payment by numbers as the outcome is not considered. NHS hospitals then compete with their neighbours and any community services offering the same 'product line' (e.g. endoscopy) for business from local or more distant PCTs and GP commissioning groups.

The government wishes to increase *patient choice* and other health care providers, principally the private sector but also voluntary organizations are being encouraged to compete with NHS providers. Thus a PCT may choose to buy knee replacement surgery from the local DGH, a private hospital, or an NHS national centre, e.g. the Royal National Orthopaedic Hospital. As the 'market' develops, the concern is that easy elective surgery will be creamed off into the private sector leaving the NHS with complex cases and emergencies – both of which will include a disproportionate number of older people. Above all, elderly people want a dependable local service.

General practitioners

In the UK every person is registered with a GP. The GP was the first point of contact for all NHS services, but a number of services can now be accessed directly, e.g. self-referral to physiotherapy, walk-in centres, calling NHS Direct for advice. This increases patient choice but care may become more fragmented. If multidisciplinary care is to succeed in the community setting, it is essential that the GP becomes the effective leader of the team. A good GP needs

- A wide knowledge of both medicine and the scope of the skills of other team members.
- Comprehensive past records and current information about the patient's problems and treatment.
- A friendly and approachable manner so that neither elderly patients nor their carers (formal or informal) are deterred from seeking help.
- Ready access to hospital-based specialists' help and advice.

GPs who wish to demonstrate their special expertise with older patients can take the Diploma of Geriatric Medicine examination of the Royal College of Physicians. They can take on extra responsibilities as a GP with a special interest in older people.

Opportunistic case finding and anticipatory care

During any consultation, there is an opportunity to pick up other health or social problems and look ahead. The GP contract ensures that the practice is paid for a number of specific quality points (QOF or Quality and Outcomes Framework). GP practices usually have very well-developed IT systems and the opportunities for paid prevention are flagged to GPs on screen. Some practices are developing registers of 'Vulnerable Older People'.

Potentially preventable diseases in old age

- Seasonal influenza – annual vaccination.
- Pneumococcal pneumonia – 5-yearly vaccination
- Multi-infarct dementia and stroke by treatment of high BP and anticoagulation for atrial fibrillation.
- Osteoporosis by achieving good peak bone mass in adult life and continuing to exercise.
- Ischaemic heart disease by avoidance of tobacco and promotion of exercise and 'Mediterranean' diet.
- Alcoholic dementia, heart failure, pancreatitis and cirrhosis, by sticking to safe numbers of units.
- Obesity, with its effect on osteoarthritis and carbohydrate metabolism.
- Type 2 diabetes, by maintaining ideal body weight and regular walking.

- Diverticular disease by increasing dietary fibre.
- COPD and bronchogenic carcinoma; risks reduced by avoiding tobacco.
- Dietary deficiency states.
- Iatrogenic disease.

Community nursing staff

An increasing number of nurses work in the community, outside hospitals and GP surgeries. They are employed by the PCT, GP practices or the voluntary sector. They include district nurses, a plethora of disease or system-specific specialist nurses, e.g. for heart failure, COPD/asthma, Parkinson's disease, continence, stoma specialists, palliative care nursing (Macmillan) and advice (Marie Curie). Many have prescribing rights. A recent concept is that of the community matron. This was based on an American model; in that different health care economy, it was an effective way of case managing older complex patients. As is often the case when government dictates health policy, the system was rolled out before evidence that it worked here and it probably does not!

Much of the total time of these nurses is devoted to the care of elderly people. They provide:
- Treatment, e.g. injections, enemas and dressings.
- Specialist care, e.g. stoma management and continence advice.
- Liaison with other services.
- Hands-on nursing (mainly supervising health care assistants).

Community psychiatric nurses

Community psychiatric nurses (CPNs) are registered mental health nurses based in community mental health teams of the Old Age Psychiatry service. They work mainly with patients with depression and dementia:
- To support the patients and carers.
- To monitor progress.
- To liaise with other services.

Hospital care of older patients

This can take the following forms:
1 Outpatient care, i.e. accident and emergency attendance and outpatient clinics.

2 Acute inpatient care.

3 Intermediate care (IC)/rehabilitation (see below).

4 Long-term care (see above).

Outpatient care

Accident/emergency department

Because of their liability to accidents, and the sudden onset of illness, the elderly are frequent users of the accident and emergency (A & E) department. Their management in such departments is difficult and the outcome may be sub-optimal for several reasons:

1 Elderly patients are often unable to give an account of themselves owing to impaired consciousness, confusion or dementia, communication difficulties (speech, hearing impairment), anxiety or fear.

2 Their problems are frequently multiple and complex.

3 They are often unaccompanied.

4 Their accident or illness is often a consequence of long-term neglect or lack of support.

5 They are more likely than most patients to require transport back home.

An overnight ward as part of A & E may allow sufficient time for the elderly to regain their equilibrium and for intermediate care in the community to be organized and thereby facilitate discharge with enhanced post-discharge support. The Department of Medicine for the Elderly should have sufficient staff to provide an immediate 24 h per day expert advisory service to their local A & E department.

Outpatient department

Irrespective of age, all appropriate patients have a right to be referred to any specialist clinic.

• Frail elderly patients are more likely to require assistance with transport to, and within, the hospital.

• All clinics should be user-friendly for elderly patients; e.g. appropriate seating (chairs with arms enable older people to get up independently), effective arrangements for deaf or partially sighted patients and wheelchair-users in the waiting area, a working communicator in the clinic room and variable height couches. Help with dressing and undressing is likely to be needed.

• Complex patients with multiple pathology are best managed in specialist geriatric clinics, supported where necessary by organ-specific specialists.

• Follow-up clinics where necessary should be held near to the patient's home, e.g. GP surgery or community hospital and not necessarily at the DGH.

Acute inpatient care

During the last 20 years, the acute bed numbers in British hospitals have been reduced by 2% annually. At the same time, admissions have risen by 3.5–5%. The elderly are the greatest users of hospital beds (65% of inpatients are over 65 years of age). Occupancy rates have always been high and often reach 97%. The system has only continued to function by the steady reduction in the length of stay for each patient including the elderly.

Most admissions are considered appropriate while between 1% and 6% being deemed not so. Inappropriate admissions may be higher among older patients, perhaps, up to 20%, especially in the very old. However, the rates of inappropriate admissions are very variable and depend on the quality of local general practice and the availability of alternative forms of care.

Reasons that expose elderly people to higher hospital admission rates are:

1 Pathology, both acute and chronic.

2 Living alone and social disadvantage.

3 Polypharmacy.

4 High accident/fall rate.

Intensive case management of older patients with chronic disease is designed to reduce admission (e.g. by identifying deteriorating cardiac failure before admission is necessary), and if admission is needed, faster discharge should be expedited by better, flexible care in the community.

Hospital hazards

The acute hospital is a dangerous place for frail elderly people. This is not a reason for depriving them of access, but should act as a stimulus to improving the safety of patients through better hospital design, improved staffing levels and mix, and improving standards of cleanliness and catering.

• Up to 50% of deaths of elderly patients in hospital may be precipitated by poor prescribing.

- Of all hospital inpatients, 10% suffer from cross-infections, especially MRSA. This rate is highest in frail elderly people.
- Broad-spectrum antibiotics may precipitate bowel overgrowth by *Clostridium difficile* and the resulting diarrhoea that may have fatal consequences.
- Falls are common because of impaired function in the patient or hospital design and inadequate staff supervision. The situation is often made worse by the inappropriate use of various forms of restraint (both physical and pharmacological).
- Patients who are malnourished on admission may deteriorate further in their nutritional status during their hospital stay owing to inappropriate catering and feeding arrangements.
- Dependency may be encouraged by poor staff attitudes and practices.
- Elderly patients are not always given appropriate priority when investigations are needed. Delays can be very detrimental. Sophisticated techniques may be more appropriate because of the elderly patient's inability to cope with demanding and invasive techniques as well as their fitter and younger counterparts.
- Surgery is more dangerous, especially if delegated to junior surgeons and anaesthetists.
- Malnutrition hampers surgical recovery.
- Ignoring pre- and post-operative medical conditions compromises the success of essential surgery.
- Post-operative complications are more common and more serious.
- Lack of appropriate community services and/or accommodation may delay discharge. Up to 70,000 patients are trapped in this way in UK hospitals at any one time. These inappropriately labelled bed-blockers or delayed discharges continue to be exposed to all of the above dangers and occupy about 6% of acute hospital beds.

As the NHS moves to a more financially driven model, delays in hospital at all ages are being measured in a new way. For each category of diagnosis, there is a predicted length of time needed in hospital. This is known as the trim point. If the patient stays in longer, these extra days are termed 'outlyer' bed days.

The Department of Medicine for the Elderly

This should provide the ideal setting for the medical and nursing management of frail elderly patients with multiple and complex problems. It should be based within the DGH, but with outreach facilities in community hospitals, the community itself and care homes. In addition, it should provide advice and support for other hospital departments caring for elderly patients, especially A & E, orthopaedic surgery and psychiatry.

Admission to a department of geriatric medicine should hasten and not limit access to other specialist opinions, such as cardiology, neurology, etc.

Mental health services for older people

These are provided by departments of old age psychiatry that are usually based in secondary care but do much of their work in the community. Psychiatry operates an age cut-off; once a patient with a psychiatric problem reaches 65, they 'graduate' from the adult service to the old age service and new patients presenting after that age go straight to the old age service. The old age psychiatrist leads a multidisciplinary team comprising specialist nurses, therapists, psychologists and social workers or case managers. Patients are usually assessed at home by one of the team, and are usually managed at home with ongoing support, not least because so many beds have been cut in this sector.

Intermediate care

Intermediate care (IC) is the umbrella term for services that sit between primary care and the DGH and are designed to be therapeutic, in contrast with care provision. IC is described in Standard 3 of the National Service Framework (see below). It covers many aspects of the management of frail elderly patients. It is intended to help maintain elderly people at home and to avoid hospital admission by intensifying care provision at times of need (e.g. an acute minor illness), to aid recovery by the provision by rehabilitation services, to assist the discharge of elderly patients from hospital through active rehabilitation programmes and to enhance the domiciliary support at the time of discharge (and is in danger of being all things to all men).

Intermediate care therefore has a role in community care, i.e. enhanced provision, and also in community hospital care in the form of rehabilitation and step-down care. This latter form of care is envisaged as a less intense, more user-friendly, less clinical, more domestic provision of inpatient services. In many ways, it replaces what was previously described as slow-stream hospital rehabilitation. Some of the provision may be nurse-led, moving away from the doctor-led medical model. However, those receiving IC are likely to be very frail and vulnerable to repeated episodes of deterioration in their health, and the input of geriatricians is essential.

Day hospitals

These are units that provide day treatment to patients living in their own homes. The physically frail attend units run by medicine for the elderly services; if mental health problems are paramount, the patient attends a service run by old age psychiatry. Transport has always been problematic. However, day hospitals are capable of providing many of the services available to inpatients, i.e. diagnosis, investigation, procedures, e.g. blood transfusion, multidisciplinary assessment and rehabilitation. Many units got bogged down providing long-term respite. This resulted in a reputation for 'custodial' care, which led to the demise of many day hospitals. Some units survived by rebadging themselves as 'Day rehabilitation units'. If money is ever really diverted back into the community, the day hospital may be due for a renaissance as it was successful in providing 'intermediate care' before the term was invented; a method of avoiding admission, shortening hospital stay and providing post-discharge support.

Social care for older people

Most elderly people wish to continue to live in their own homes. This aspiration is supported by

Table 2.2 Estimated numbers of clients 65 and over receiving services 2004–2005.

Domiciliary care	No. of recipients
Day care	135,000
Meals	165,000
Professional support	216,000
Equipment and adaptations	376,000
Home care	483,000

the government but good community services are not a cheap option, and the services are often fragmented, inadequate and under-funded or inefficient depending on your viewpoint.

The local authority was the agency responsible for assessing and purchasing domiciliary and community social care for residents, but in many areas social care and health care have merged. Over 95% of the elderly population live independently, but about 10% of these need formal community services in order to maintain their independence within their own homes (Table 2.2). Community-based services were provided to about 1.025 million clients aged 65 and over in 2004–5, accounting for 84% of all older clients receiving services. An estimated 1.23 million (71%), of those receiving services as part of a package of care were aged 65 and over.

When the person stays in their own home what types of care can be provided?

24-h care

This is extremely expensive. At least two carers are needed to cover shifts and holidays. Individuals may pay for this privately or it is occasionally paid for as NHS CC.

Regular visits for care

Domiciliary care services are the commonest way frail people are enabled to stay at home. Such care can be arranged and paid for privately and is limited only by the financial means of the individual and the availability of suitable carers in the locality. Carers can be found through care agencies or by private advertisement. Caution is needed as the clients are vulnerable and all agencies should carry out Criminal Records Bureau checks. If an individual wishes to have statutory care, their needs must be assessed by a care manager and a care package is drawn up. The care may be commissioned from in-house staff (social services or PCT), or the private sector through agencies. Care is now generally provided by generic care assistants who will perform a range of tasks. A package might consist of a visit (30 min) to get the client up, washed, dressed and breakfast, a lunchtime visit (15 min) to heat the pre-delivered frozen meal and an evening visit (20 min) to get the client back to bed. Once the client can no longer use the toilet independently between visits, or make themselves a hot drink, things become precarious, but many such individuals prefer to remain at home. If they cannot transfer with the help of one person, 'double-up' care may be needed (two carers) and such patients will usually be padded up (incontinence) and sat in their chair until the next visit (risk of pressure sores). In most areas in England and Wales this type of care is means tested.

In the community care survey 2005, the average number of contact hours per household was 10.1 in a week. In 2004, the average number of contact hours was 9.4. This suggests that more intensive services are being provided for a smaller number of service users, continuing the trend seen over the last 10 years. Statutory services have had to focus on frailer clients as funding has not kept pace with the increasing numbers of old people. If clients need help with cleaning and shopping – the old role of the home-help, rather than personal care – they are usually expected to pay for this privately, so good value services such as that run in some areas by Age Concern are much in demand.

Meals-on-wheels service

This provides clients with hot meals in their own home. Meals are provided at mid-day. There are practical problems in providing meals that remain appetizing and nutritious after delays caused by storage and delivery; some clients love them, others throw them away or are too muddled to eat them. A variety of special meals, e.g. vegetarian, diabetic, kosher and halal may be available. Some areas have moved to a system of delivering frozen ready meals. The client needs a freezer and a microwave and reasonable cognitive function to learn what may be an entirely new method of heating food. Currently in the UK, more than 26 million meals are provided by this service each year and about 3% of elderly people benefit, rising to 12% in the over-85s.

Luncheon clubs

These are centres where meals are provided, usually at subsidized prices, run by either the local authority or voluntary organizations. They provide meals to 3% of the elderly population, i.e. similar provision to meals-on-wheels service. Frequency of meal provision from luncheon clubs is less than that provided by the meals-on-wheels service – usually just once or twice weekly – but companionship is offered in addition to food. Transport is often a limiting factor.

Day centres

These are very varied and may be run by the local authority or voluntary groups but must not be confused with day hospitals. Staff may be trained (social workers, therapists) or untrained or a combination of both. A charge for attendance is usually made and transport may be provided. About 5% of elderly people attend day centres.

Day centres aim

- To combat loneliness.
- To provide diversional activity and recreation.
- To provide a meal and other comforts.
- To relieve carers.
- To disseminate health education, e.g. about falls risk.
- To encourage activity, e.g. regular exercise and balance groups.
- To introduce clients to other forms of care.

Respite care

This is the temporary provision of a bed, usually in a care home, for frail patients with chronic irremediable diseases, to give the informal carers a well-earned break. The service is organized by social services/the PCT and is means-tested. It may smooth the path to eventual permanent placement, e.g. for a person with dementia. However, periods of respite care often have an adverse effect on the recipients – especially if they are unable to comprehend the reasons for such respite care. Respite care should not be confused with crisis intervention, i.e. when a supporting system suddenly collapses, nor should it be considered as top-up rehabilitation, although there is minimal provision for the latter. However, because of the bed shortages and pressures if a frail person suddenly deteriorates in a non-specific way (see Chapter 3), they may be put in a respite bed only to be admitted to the DGH 3 days later with severe pneumonia.

Specialist equipment

A range of traditional equipment can be provided, e.g. bed and toilet rails, bath board, handling belts, a commode and even hospital beds, a hoist and wheelchair. Lifeline pendant alarms enable the wearer to summon help. Even more expensive equipment such as stair lifts can be fitted and modifications made to the house, e.g. doorways widened for wheelchairs, a level access shower; there are often delays and wrangling over who pays.

Telecare is the use of electronic technology to monitor and assist people to maintain independence in their own environment. A telecare service can monitor three components: safety and security; physiological parameters and activity. Devices include video-monitoring, fall detectors, sensors to monitor activity (a pressure mat activated as the person gets out of bed can turn on the light, detectors monitoring the fridge and front door can be used to monitor feeding and wandering etc.), wet bed alerts can summon a night carer, automatic taps prevent floods, and everyone should have smoke alarms.

Roving warden schemes

These are area-based and support a number of older people living in their original accommodation.

Regulation of health and social care

Currently this is the responsibility of the Healthcare Commission and the Commission for Social Care Inspection. It is planned that these will merge in 2008, together with responsibilities for mental health care.

Who cares?

Paid carers provide the care described above but 'informal carers' provide the majority of care. These are the most important members of the caring workforce. They are unpaid, untrained, but devoted and effective. Although the generations tend to live apart, there continues to be frequent contact within a family and almost 50% of elderly people living alone have regular daily contact with a family member. The bulk of community support is provided by family and friends – the following points are relevant to the situation within the UK:

• The proportion of dependants, i.e. children under 16 years, men over 65 years and women over 60 years of age in the community, has not increased during this century (Table 2.3).

• There are now more dependent elderly people in the community than dependent children. However, consider how much support goes into helping people look after children in comparison with older dependants.

• It is calculated that in the UK there are 6 million informal carers.

Table 2.3 Percentage of dependants in the community, i.e. pensioners and children.

Year	%
1901	41
1951	37
1981	40
1991	39
2001	40

• Most carers are women (60%) and over half of 'housewives' can expect to be called upon at some time to help an elderly and infirm person.

• Many carers are themselves pensioners. The mean age of carers of confused elderly people is 61 years. There is also a high social cost to informal carers in England and Wales. In 2001, 342,032 people aged 65 and over provided 50 h or more of unpaid care per week.

• Social services have a duty to assess carers if this is requested; between October 2004 and March 2005, 54,000 carer's assessments were carried out in England where the carer was 75+.

Strategies to improve care of older people

The **National Service Framework for Older People** (NSF OP), 2001, is one of a series of 'frameworks' and was prepared by a multidisciplinary committee set up by the government to improve standards of care within the statutory services for older people.

Recommendations of the NSF OP

• Standard 1 – routing out age discrimination. NHS services will be provided regardless of age on the basis of clinical need alone. Social care services will not use age in their eligibility criteria or policies to restrict access to available services. Ageism is, however, often covert rather than explicit.

• Standard 2 – person centred care. NHS and social care services will treat older people as individuals and enable them to make choices about their own care. This is achieved through the single assessment process, integrated commissioning arrangements and integrated provision of services including community equipment and continence services.

• Standard 3 – intermediate care. Older people will have access to a new range of IC at home or in designated care settings to promote their independence by providing enhanced services from the NHS and local councils to prevent unnecessary hospital admission, effective rehabilitation services to enable early discharge from hospital and to prevent premature or unnecessary admission to long-term residential care.

• Standard 4 – general hospital care. Older people's care in hospital is delivered through appropriate specialist care and by hospital staff who have the right set of skills to meet their needs.

• Standard 5 – stroke. The NHS will take action to prevent stroke, working in partnership with other agencies where appropriate.

• Standard 6 – falls. The NHS, working in partnership with councils, will take action to prevent falls and reduce resultant fractures or other injuries in their populations of older people.

• Standard 7 – mental health in older people. Older people who have mental health problems will have access to integrated mental health services provided by the NHS and councils to ensure effective diagnosis, treatment and support for them and their carers.

• Standard 8 – the promotion of health and active life in older age. The health and well-being of older people is promoted through a coordinated programme of action led by the NHS with support from councils.

A New Ambition for Old Age (2006) is the second phase of the NSF and concentrates on dignity, joined-up care and healthy ageing.

Needs of carers

Recognition
  • By family and friends.
  • By professionals.
  • By the state.

Support
  • Financial.
  • Social.
  • Psychological.
  • Professional.
  • Self-help groups.

Respite
  • Short periods (e.g. day care).
  • Long periods – intermittent admission to care.
  • Sitting services (e.g. Crossroads).
  • Immediate in emergencies.

Information
  • About the patient's illness.
  • About available services.

Financial allowances that can be claimed by some UK pensioners

Two million pensioners live in poverty (before housing costs are considered) where poverty is defined as a household income <60% median for all households.

Pensions are very complicated and always changing. Know the basics, look on the Age Concern website for details and always suggest that patients get advice from Citizens Advice Bureau, Help the Aged or Age Concern.

1 Basic state pension plus Christmas bonus plus winter fuel payments. The basic state pension is provided if sufficient national insurance contributions were made during working life. In 2006–2007, a single person's pension was £84.25; a married couple could receive £134.75–168.50 depending on national insurance contributions. Graduated or additional contributions may be made towards the pension if appropriate contributions had been made in earlier years.

2 Income support – savings must be minimal. Value of home not included, but any other properties must be taken into account. Grounds for possible extra money – usually for people receiving income support – is given below:

- Age over 80 (25p)!
- Blindness.
- Mortgage interest.
- Water rates.
- Ground rent and service charges.
- House insurance and repairs.
- Special diet.
- Bereavement.
- Special laundry, e.g. for incontinence.
- Heating, e.g. cold weather payments and help with insulation work (Warm front grants).
- Hospital fares and other special transport costs.
- Board and lodging for residential care and NHs.
- Council tax.

3 Social fund (community care grants). Loans made for replacement of clothing, repairs to home, redecoration, bedding and furniture, etc.

4 Housing benefit from the local authority housing department for rent.

5 Attendance allowance (day or night allowances) routinely only paid for disabilities of greater duration than 6 months, unless there is a prognosis of <6 months when there is no qualifying period. This is non-means tested, paid to the claimant and is probably the most useful additional benefit. The client must need help with personal care.

6 Extra money for carers,

- Invalid care allowance for a carer who is a low wage earner and who provides more than 35 h of care per week.
- Home responsibility protection to protect pension rights of carers.

7 Death grant to help pay for funerals if extra financial help is required. It must be requested before the funeral is carried out.

8 Concessions are available for all pensioners for bus and rail travel and entry to places of entertainment – but local variations in generosity and age qualifications.

9 All pensioners over the age of 75 are now entitled to a free television licence.

Further information

Department of Health home page: http://www.dh.gov.uk/en/Home

New steps in implementing the NSF, a new ambition for old age
http://www.dh.gov.uk/PublicationsAndStatistics/Publications/PublicationPolicyAndGuidance/DH_4133941.

Age Concern website: http://www.ageconcern.org/.

Community care statistics from the NHS and social care information centre: http://www.ic.nhs.uk/pubs/commcare05adultengsum/NationalSummary2004-05v4.doc/file.

Community care statistics for supported residents in care: ttp://www.ic.nhs.uk/pubs/comcaresrae2005/ICpublication_view.

GP Quality and Outcomes Framework (2004): http://www.dh.gov.uk/assetRoot/04/08/86/93/04088693.pdf.

Laing and Buisson data on long-term care sector: http://www.laingbuisson.co.uk/StatisticsInformation/LongTermCare/tabid/71/Default.aspx.

Chapter 3

Special features of medicine in the elderly

The ageing of populations

As explained in Chapters 1 and 2, developed countries experienced a large increase in the proportion of elderly citizens during the 20th century, particularly during its closing decade. Reasons for this include falling fertility rates and falling death rates at all ages but particularly in infancy and early childhood, owing to improved living standards (housing, hygiene, nutrition and heating). The increasing number of very elderly people is, however, partly owing to the improvements in medicine in adult life. Many underdeveloped countries are also experiencing a growth in older people, sometimes exaggerated by the loss of the younger generation because of HIV infection.

Blessing or curse?

Increasing longevity sounds like a blessing – but that depends on whether the extra years are years of good health and activity. Does the 'rectangularization of the survival curve' lead to a 'compression of morbidity' into the final months of life or to a prolonged period of disability and dependency? One recent estimate gave a 65-year-old man an average of 8 further years of active life followed by 6 years of significant disability, and a woman 10 years and 9 years, respectively. At age 75, these

figures were, respectively, 4 years and 4 years for a man, and 6.5 years and 4.5 years for a woman.

The ageing cell

Some cells (neurons, renal and myocardial) do not divide and have to last a lifetime, although there is a decline in their numbers. Normal human embryonic fibroblasts have a fixed capacity to divide around 50 times, but those from mature subjects have a reduced capacity for reduplication. This may be due to telomerase inactivation in somatic cells (unlike the germ-line) with telomere shortening, telomerase reactivation being a possible explanation for the immortality of malignant cells in culture. Other features of these cells from aged individuals include:

1 Aneuploidy (variable chromosome numbers).
2 Increased numbers of nucleoli.
3 Lipofuscin pigment granules in cytoplasm in neurons, liver, kidney and muscle.
4 Mitochondrial respiratory-chain function (energy release) less efficient in skeletal muscle.
5 Cells are more vulnerable to free-radical damage.

Ageing connective tissue

Stiffness and loss of elasticity occur because of cross-linkages (e.g. disulphide bonds) forming bridges between adjacent collagen molecules, especially in skin, elastic laminae of blood vessels, tendons and lens of eye.

Immunity and ageing

1 Thymic involution and attenuated T-cell-mediated immunity lead to reactivation of quiescent infections, such as TB and varicella. There seems to be a decline in delayed-type skin-hypersensitivity reactions to injected antigens (anergy) in many frail aged subjects.

2 Certain autoantibodies occur more frequently in old age – e.g. antiphospholipid antibodies, which are associated with vascular disease but their significance in older people is uncertain.

3 Proliferative disorders of the lymphocyte are very common.

4 Malnutrition and diabetes compound these problems.

Declining function

Many physiological parameters decline with age but the magnitude of the decline is hard to estimate. These figures are almost always based on cross-sectional rather than longitudinal studies, which will include individuals within the elderly cohort who have acquired diseases that may affect function, e.g. renal function will suffer as a result of hypertension or diabetes, or whose sedentary lifestyle in retirement has caused cardiorespiratory fitness to decline through disuse. To be attributable to ageing per se, a phenomenon must be universal, intrinsic and progressive. Watching the London Marathon will reveal many 70 or even 80+ year olds fitter than most people in their thirties and forties.

Special features of illness in older patients

Illness in older people is usually a continuum of conditions found in middle age, but the illness occurs in the context of ageing and lack of fitness, and the social situation the person is in (Figure 3.1).

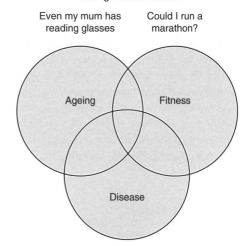

Background to disease

Even my mum has reading glasses

Could I run a marathon?

Ageing

Fitness

Disease

Figure 3.1 In an older person, the impact of the disease depends on the level of fitness and physiological ageing of the individual.

Background of ageing

Ageing changes are seen in *most organs* (go through the body in your mind), e.g. brain, special senses and peripheral nerves.

Why do ageing changes matter?
• Increased variability between individuals.
• Okay at rest, significant when stressed (e.g. fasting glucose minimally higher in elderly, but glucose levels higher after meals).
• Impaired homeostasis results in problems when the environment becomes more challenging. In extreme old age the challenge may be minimal, such as maintaining BP on standing. Some physical signs have different significance, e.g. small pupils, poor upgaze and wasting of small muscles of the hand.

Multiple pathology and aetiology

Why do old people often have several diseases?

The prevalence of many diseases increases with age (e.g. stroke, Parkinson's disease and Alzheimer's disease) so the fact that older people have several diseases may simply reflect this. Some chronic diseases have complications affecting several systems (e.g. diabetes may lead to heart, eye, kidney and nerve problems) or may predispose to other disorders (e.g. infections). Also, a risk factor may predispose the individual to several diseases (e.g. smokers are more likely to have chronic bronchitis, lung cancer, heart disease, strokes, gangrene, macular degeneration and osteoporosis). One problem may also have several causes (multiple aetiology); e.g. falls are usually multi-factorial (previous stroke + poor vision + osteoarthritis of the knees, etc.).

Different risk factors

It must not be assumed that parameters (e.g. high lipid levels) that constitute a risk factor in the young carry the same risk in the elderly in the absence of positive evidence. An 85-year-old person with a cholesterol level of 8 mmol/L presumably has 'protective' genes and so the significance of this finding is not the same as in a 40-year-old person.

Different susceptibility to disease

This is more of a theoretical possibility than a practical consideration. However, TB may be commoner (reasons may include socio-economic factors, prior exposure, changes in the immune system, etc.).

Different differential diagnosis

Although the range of possible diagnoses may be similar at any age, age is important in determining what is most likely. Fits and jaundice that are the commonest causes will be different in the neonate, child, young adult and old person.

Altered response to disease

Many older people present in exactly the same way as middle-aged people, e.g. crushing central chest pain in a myocardial infarct. However, this is not always the case and this makes diagnosis in the frail older person a diagnostic challenge. There may be:
- Missing symptoms, e.g. pain, fever and thirst.
- Missing signs, e.g. neck stiffness.

Finally, non-specific presentation is common. The 'geriatric giants' – the big 'I's – are common features of illness in old age:
- Intellectual failure (acute or chronic confusion).
- Incontinence (if this is new, why?).
- Immobility ('off her feet').
- Instability (falls).
- Iatrogenic disease (see the section titled 'Pharmacological Treatment).
- Inability to look after oneself (functional decline or in an analogy to paediatrics, 'failure to thrive').

All of these vague and dull-sounding clinical pictures, often labelled 'social problem' in the medical record, are almost never because of social problems and could be because of a huge range of serious and treatable conditions – if you look – e.g. myocardial infarct, stroke, Parkinson's disease (PD), and so on.

Consequences of immobility

These include dehydration, incontinence, pressure sores, deep vein thrombosis, and so on, and often complicate the presenting condition.

Low expectations

Why do old people sometimes present so late in their illness?

Older people may have poor expectations of the health care system, fuelled by friends and family and sometimes, sadly, by previous experience of health care professionals. 'What do you expect at your age?' is a remark familiar to many. The problem may be compounded by lack of medical understanding, so that urinary incontinence and swollen ankles are assumed to be normal.

Social problems

Old age is a time of loss (family, friends, income, housing, mobility, independence and life itself). This is one aspect of medicine for older people that can be sad. There may be practical solutions – how will the problems affect the patient? However, often what are most appreciated are support and a little of your time to hear about how things were.

Advantages and disadvantages of 'labels'

Be circumspect before labelling people. Doctors spend a great deal of time attaching diagnostic labels to people. This is part of the job; the label usually helps the patient to understand what is causing their symptoms and helps the clinicians to manage the condition. However, sometimes labels are unhelpful – a 93-year-old woman with impaired glucose tolerance labelled 'diabetic' may be refused Christmas cake in her residential home. It is very difficult to shake off an incorrect label, and so if in doubt, remain descriptive, e.g. 'breathless with shadow on CXR', pending further investigation.

The importance of functional assessment and rehabilitation

Expensive and technically successful intervention is of limited value if the patient does not recover the ability to enjoy a worthwhile quality of life. Overall assessment should include a comprehensive list of medical problems and their prioritization in terms of threat to quality and quantity of life [an assessment of cognitive function, evaluation of functional abilities, some idea of the social background ('ecological niche') and who is there to do tasks for the patient when he or she is unable to do them for him or herself]. It will take an older person longer to recover strength and function after a severe systemic illness – this may be obvious to the reader, but is not always obvious to patient, family and medical attendant.

Rehabilitation

Rehabilitation is defined as the restoration of the individual to his or her fullest physical, mental and social capability. It takes several forms:

1 Restoration to full activity after a severe illness (e.g. abdominal surgery, and myocardial infarction).
2 Restoration of maximum achievable function following a specific impairment (e.g. stroke and fractured femoral neck).
3 Facilitating the achievement of as much independence as possible despite continuing impairment (e.g. Parkinson's disease, amputation, partially recovered stroke and hip disease).

Rehabilitation can take place in a variety of settings (see box). It is an active process and it is important that the multi-disciplinary team, (see box) including the patient and carer, share common objectives. Regular goal-setting meetings are useful. If the patient is not progressing as well as anticipated, it is important to look for barriers that may be interfering with the process. These include

---

The rehabilitation team

Patient.
Family.
Nurses.
Rehabilitation professions (physiotherapists, occupational therapists, speech therapists).
Doctor.
Clinical psychologist.
Dietician.
Chiropodist.
Appliance officer.
Social worker.
Voluntary workers.

Rehabilitation settings

Acute hospital ward (includes orthopaedic wards).
Rehabilitation ward in acute hospital.
Rehabilitation ward in community hospital.
Stroke units, wherever situated.
Outpatient therapy departments.
Geriatric day hospital.
Psychiatric counterparts of the above.
Primary-care premises.
Residential/nursing homes.
Community groups, e.g. stroke clubs, keep-fit classes.
Patient's own home (e.g. domiciliary therapy, patient's and carer's own efforts).

---

depression, uncontrolled pain and hidden agendas, e.g. 'if I improve, I will be a burden to them'.

Rehabilitation from acute illness

Hospital admission is often required, not for specific investigations or medication that cannot be administered at home, but because the weakness associated with a chest infection or heart disease renders patients unable to attend to their bodily needs (nutrition, fluid intake, bowel, bladder, hygiene, etc.) unassisted. He or she may feel too unwell to get out of bed for a day or two. Unless there is adequate support at home, admission needs to be arranged without delay; otherwise pressure sores, contractures, constipation, incontinence and loss of confidence are inevitable and will necessitate protracted rehabilitation. Remobilization is achieved by suitable exercises (passive, assisted, resisted), combined with functional exercise, such as transfers, sitting to standing and walking. Activities of daily living (ADL) abilities are assessed and various items of equipment may be deployed to facilitate independence. An attempt at quantitative measurement of function is provided by the Barthel scale (see Appendix 2). Following discharge, the able-bodied may consider positive measures to promote physical fitness.

Even if there is irremediable impairment, it may be possible to reduce disability or handicap.

- *Impairment* loss or abnormality of structure or function, e.g. weak leg and arm following stroke.
- *Disability* the resulting loss of ability to perform an activity in the normal manner, e.g. a diminished ability to walk.
- *Handicap* the ensuing disadvantage in terms of fulfilment of the individual's role, e.g. unable to cook and do the housework or participate in leisure activities, and so on.

Principles of rehabilitation

1 Rehabilitation is needed after all illnesses not just after stroke or fracture, etc.

2 A multi-disciplinary activity including the patient and the patient's informal carers.

3 Essential to know what the patient could do before the current illness.

3 Full assessment of the patient's problems is required before the process starts.

4 Goals must be realistic with defined end points.

5 Logical step-by-step approach to achieve the set goals.

6 A continuous process – 'every activity is a therapeutic opportunity', i.e. rehabilitation does not just occur when face to face with a therapist.

7 Rehabilitation should never really end as maintenance is required if the achieved improvements are to be retained.

8 Rehabilitation can take place in a variety of settings depending on circumstances.

Rehabilitation is not always the most appropriate way to manage severe disability. A palliative approach is sometimes the best and kindest option.

Barriers to successful rehabilitation

- Global impairment of higher cerebral function.
- Poor motivation (patient or carers).
- Depression.
- Communication difficulties.
- Sensory deprivation.
- Associated pathology (arthritis, heart failure).
- Pressure sores, contractures.
- Loss of body image, sensory ataxia, disordered visuospatial perception.
- Swallowing difficulty.
- Unrealistic expectations.
- Effects of disease, injury, and so on.

Ethical problems

The whole area of denial of access to high-class care versus overaggressive and futile intervention – discriminating ageism versus compassionate ageism – is a major minefield and one of the fascinations of geriatric medicine. See also Chapter 16.

Examination of the aged patient – things to look out for

Gait

- Aided or unaided?
- Foot drop?
- Shuffling or striding? Stable or unstable?
- Difficulty up/down from chair?
- Parkinsonian or multi-infarct?

Face

- Parkinsonian (the 'disconcerting reptilian gaze', immobility, flexed posture).
- Depression.
- Hypothyroidism, anaemia, vitiligo.
- Angular stomatitis (often due to ill-fitting dentures).
- Orofacial dyskinesia.
- Ptosis – symmetrical ('senile') or unilateral (eye surgery or Horner's).
- Basal-cell carcinoma.
- Facial palsy.

Joint disease

- The stiff neck.
- The tentative handshake of rotator-cuff atrophy, difficulty getting in/out of sleeves.
- Stiff hips/knees.
- Kyphosis and protuberant abdomen suggestive of osteoporosis.

Self-neglect

- Dirty hands/face/body.
- Dirty clothing, evidence of incontinence.
- Unshaven, hair unkempt.
- Neglected nails.

Nutrition

- Obesity.
- Protein–energy undernutrition – compare weight with previous records; signs of recent weight loss or extreme cachexia.
- Hydration.

Conversation

- Dyspnoea?
- Good account of circumstances?
- Plausible, with obvious lacunae?
- Mood?
- Speech – dysphasia, dysarthria, dysphonia?
- Emotional lability.

Formal examination

- Extrasystoles – common and seldom significant.
- Neglected breast cancer.
- Displaced apex beat – due to chest deformity which also affects traditional radiation of mumurs.
- Peripheral pulses – palpate and auscultate.
- Abdomen – ribs tend to sit over pelvis, so hard to ballot kidneys, distended bladder and faecal impaction.
- Defective up-gaze – common, dubious significance.
- Ankle jerks – usually present – plantar strike often the best technique.

Pharmacological treatment: special considerations

The elderly consume most drugs (prescribed or over-the-counter). The oldest 15% of the population receive 40% of all drug prescriptions. Older people are:
- More sensitive to drugs (weight, renal function, etc). The estimated glomerular filtration rate (eGFR) can be looked up easily on the net.
- More susceptible to side-effects and adverse effects.
- More likely to have side-effects that have serious sequelae.

Pharmacokinetics and pharmacodynamics

Pharmacokinetics (what the body does to the drug) and pharmacodynamics (what the drug does to the body) are both affected by ageing. Examples include:
- Slower gastric emptying.
- Increased ratio of adipose to lean tissue (increased volume of distribution for fat-soluble drugs, e.g. diazepam).
- Reduced plasma albumin.
- Altered liver metabolism – affects first pass (chlormethiazole and paracetamol).
- Reduced renal clearance (very important when a drug excreted by the kidney has a narrow therapeutic index, e.g. digoxin).

• Increased receptor sensitivity (psychoactive drugs and warfarin).

When problems arise there are often many causes

Example

Nellie Smith does not get out much because of her arthritic knees. She is prescribed a non-steroidal anti-inflammatory drug (NSAID):
• Decides indigestion is normal at her age (expectations).
• Has a haematemesis (more prone to side-effects).
• Collapses (impaired homeostasis, exacerbated by her frusemide).
• Fractures her hip (co-existing osteoporosis).
• Is not found until the next day (social factors – lives alone).
• Is admitted but has complications (need for speed to avoid complications of immobility).
• Antibiotics are prescribed (iatrogenic – third-generation cephalosporins should be avoided if possible).
• Develops *Clostridium difficile* diarrhoea from which she may die….
Was the NSAID indicated initially?

Multiple pathology means multiple therapy

Older people on several drugs are:
• More likely to experience side-effects, drug interactions and adverse drug reactions.
• Likely to have problems with concordance, especially if confused.
• Often on a drug to treat the side-effects of another!

Reviewing the drugs – repeat prescriptions

Review your patient's problem list and prioritize the treatable. The patient is usually on many drugs already. For each drug consider:
• If the likely benefit outweighs the risk? (e.g. Mr Roland, 74 years old, is on warfarin for **stroke risk reduction secondary to atrial Gbrillation (AG)** has dementia, is prone to falls and is found to have an unexpected INR of 7.2: stop the warfarin and you may save his life.)

• Still indicated? (Oxybutinin, sulphonylurea, etc. are often continued with little evidence of efficacy.)
• 'Nicest' drug for the job (e.g. clarithromycin has fewer gastric side-effects than erythromycin)?
• Is the drug causing the symptoms (e.g. nausea or confusion due to codeine; frusemide and fludrocortisone are an illogical combination)?
• Could a single agent replace two (e.g. ACE inhibitor for hypertension with CCF)?
• Is the formulation/route of administration the best (e.g. syrups and patches may help) ?
• Timings appropriate (e.g. once-a-day or twice-a-day options aid adherence for the patient or visiting carers) ?
• Aids to administration (e.g. spacer for inhalers, no childproof tops)?
• Aids to adherence (e.g. dosette box.)?
• Regular or 'as required'? (Analgesics are usually best given on a regular basis.)
• Does the patient understand the medications and any precautions? (Supply written information and record advice in the notes.)
• Cheapest (if there are equivalents e.g. proton-pump inhibitors)?

Should a new drug be started?

• With the aim of cure or disease modification, symptom control, or primary or secondary prevention.
• Start low, go slow, but increase the dose until in the therapeutic range or side-effects develop.
• Give a drug for long enough time before deciding it is ineffective, e.g. antidepressants.
• Where the aim is prevention, consider the overall burden of pathology and drugs, but avoid therapeutic nihilism.

How many drugs are reasonable?

Cardiac guidelines in many countries, including NICE Guidelines for treatment after MI in the UK, recommend multiple drugs:
• Beta-blocker.
• Aspirin.
• Clopidogrel for a month after STEMI, a year after NSTEMI.

- ACE inhibitor and perhaps ARB too The Candesartan in Heart Failure Assessment of Reduction in Morbidity and mortality (CHARM).
- Statin.
- With heart failure – loop diuretic and spironolactone.
- With diabetes – insulin in the acute phase, usual treatment later.
- With AF – warfarin or aspirin and dipyridamole.
- With angina – nicorandil.

Summary: the overall picture

- If there are multiple drugs, are they all essential?
- Try to avoid drugs to treat the side-effects of another drug.
- Look for potential interactions.
- If the patient has renal failure, do not rely on memory, check every drug against the list in the British National Formulary (BNF).
- The patient will change. Always review medication. Is secondary prevention still appropriate?

Surgery in elderly patients

Obligatory versus facultative

The former category includes resection of a colonic carcinoma or fixation of a hip fracture, the latter includes life-enhancing procedures, such as elective hip replacement or cataract extraction.

Emergency versus elective

At age over 75 years, the mortality for emergency surgery is 60 – 80%.

The main risk factors for elective surgical patients are:

1 Cardiac: infarction during preceding 3 months or failure.
2 Respiratory: chronic obstructive lung disease, current smoking.
3 CNS: stroke during preceding 3 months, dementia.
4 Metabolic: diabetes, steroid medication, renal failure.
5 Significantly overweight or underweight.
6 Frailty and poor mobility.

Peri-operative care

The amount that can be achieved pre-operatively depends on the urgency of surgery. For elective surgery, patients can be encouraged to stop smoking and improve their fitness (often not achievable if the surgery is for chronic pain, e.g. knee replacement). It may be possible to improve gross protein–energy undernutrition (by nasogastric tube if necessary) and optimize pre-existing drugs. Check whether the patient is on warfarin (replace with heparin if necessary) and whether other drugs should be given on the morning of surgery – it may be better to stop ACE inhibitors the day before. It is essential to correct heart failure, salt and water depletion, respiratory infection and severe anaemia. The skill of the anesthetist is as important as the surgeon in ensuring good operative outcome; frail old people are usually assessed pre-operatively by a senior anaesthetist who will decide whether general or regional anaesthesia is appropriate.

Ageing affects the pharmacokinetics and pharmacodynamics of many anaesthetic drugs. Premedication is often avoided in the very old and reduced doses are needed for many drugs. During surgery the aim is to avoid episodes of excessive hypotension after induction of anaesthesia or large blood loss, or the combination of hypertension and tachycardia after noxious stimulation. Special care is also needed to avoid pressure damage and maintain body temperature. Post-operative analgesia requires careful control to maximize pain relief with minimal sedation or respiratory depression.

Post-operative complications

1 Respiratory infection – especially high-risk subjects resulting from atelectasis due to suppression of full inspiration by pain (abdominal surgery) or sedation.
2 Confusion – commonest on day 3 or 4 and following orthopaedic rather than general surgical procedures, possibly related to cerebral fat embolism. Other causes are mentioned in Chapter 4 under acute confusional states, drugs and alcohol or their abrupt withdrawal being particularly important. Another predictable cause is hyponatraemia caused by bladder irrigation during prostatectomy.

Sensory deprivation is a risk factor, as is discomfort due to pain or bladder distension.

3 Cardiac failure (in 5–10% of surgical patients over 65 years) – sometimes due to overenthusiastic fluid replacement.

4 MI (1–4%) – half are painless – 'failure to thrive' post-operatively – comparison with a pre-operative ECG can assist the diagnosis.

5 Stroke (3% of patients over 80 years of age undergoing surgery).

6 DVT – 25–33%; it is important to follow prophylactic guidelines.

7 Pressure sores (see also Chapter 15).

Further information

Barat, I., Andreasen F. and Damsgaard E.M. (2000) The consumption of drugs by 75-year-old individuals living in their own homes. *European Journal of Clinical Pharmacology*, **56**, 501–9.

McMurdo, M.E. (2000) A healthy old age: realistic or futile goal? *British Medical Journal*, **321**, 1149–51.

NICE web site: www.nice.org.uk/nice-web

Sear, J.W. and Higham, H. (2002) Issues in the perioperative management of the elderly patient with cardiovascular disease. *Drugs & Aging*, **19**(6): 429–51.

Thomas, H.F., Sweetnam, P.M., Janchawee, B. and Luscombe, D.K. (1999) Polypharmacy among older men in South Wales. *European Journal of Clinical Pharmacology*, **55**, 411–15.

Chapter 4

Old age psychiatry

Age changes

Brain weight decreases by 20% by the age of 90 years, there is selective neuronal loss of between 5% and 50% and the cells tend to shrink. There is also a 15–20% reduction in synapses in the frontal lobes. Lipofuscin accumulates in some cells, but its significance is uncertain. Plaques and tangles are found in aged brains but seldom in middle-aged ones. Granulovacuolar degeneration can often be found in the hippocampus and occasional vascular amyloid deposits are seen in cortical blood vessels. All these changes are more pronounced in Alzheimer's disease (AD), but AD is not just exaggerated ageing.

Performance in intelligence testing, learning ability, short-term memory and reaction time tend to decline with age (see age-associated memory impairment, p. 38) but often not significantly until about the age of 75 years.

Sleep

There is a positive correlation between increasing age and complaints of poor sleep. Studies indicate that sleep becomes shorter, lighter and more broken, with greater difficulty getting back to sleep again. Stages 3 and 4 of sleep are rarely attained and periods of rapid-eye-movement sleep are also infrequent. Apnoeic episodes are commoner. The worst sleep patterns are found in patients with dementia.

Simple advice for poor sleepers

- Do not have unrealistic expectations.
- Rise at a regular and early hour.
- Maintain activity during the day – avoid daytime napping.
- Avoid coffee or tea during the evening.
- Keep the bedroom for sleeping, not watching TV, etc.
- Wind down before trying to get to sleep.
- Do not go to bed hungry.
- Take a warm milky drink in the evening.
- Do not go to bed too early.

Factors that disturb sleep patterns

- Anxiety.
- Depression.
- Pain.
- Discomfort due to constipation.
- Urgency, frequency, nocturia.
- Restless legs (pramipexole and ropinirole are licensed treatments).
- Cramps.
- Nocturnal cough or breathlessness.
- Drugs (theophylline, sympathomimetics, high dose steroids).
- Drug withdrawal (sedatives, hypnotics).

If simple corrective measures do not help, look for and treat any factors listed in the preceding box. Hypnotics are avoided if possible as elderly persons are more likely to fall e.g. if they have to get up to go to the toilet and there may be a hangover effect the next day, but if the situation is causing distress, a short course of a hypnotic may be justified.

Problem drinking

Repeated ingestion leads to dependency, physical disease or other harm. Consumption peaks at age 55 and declines thereafter. One survey has shown that 17% of people aged over 60 have a problem and 12% are heavy drinkers. The usual problem is daily dosing rather than bingeing, so this is often not apparent. For this reason, a simple screening tool like CAGE (see Appendix 3) may be useful. Older people may have particular problems with alcohol if their balance or cognition is already impaired, with obesity or malnutrition and alcohol predisposes to hypothermia. Treatment of alcoholics entails total withdrawal: delirium tremens is controlled with chlordiazepoxide (but lower doses may be needed than the 'standard' protocol). In problem drinking, it may be possible to reduce intake – check who is buying the alcohol. The Institute of Alcohol Studies produces a useful fact sheet, and Alcoholics Anonymous (AA) offers helpful support for those who find their methods acceptable.

Anxiety

Anxiety is very common in older people and may accompany depression, dementia and physical illness or may cause physical symptoms (palpitations, breathlessness, giddiness, abdominal discomfort, bowel fixation). Always consider anxiety or depression in recurrent attenders with a GP or in a hospital setting, and in rehabilitation patients who fail to make progress. Treatment is by reassurance or cognitive therapy, but if severe and amounting to panic attacks, SSRIs are the drugs of choice.

Paraphrenia (persistent delusional disorder)

This is a late-life schizophreniform paranoid psychosis in which personality and affect are well preserved and there is no thought disorder. It most often affects unmarried women who live alone, especially those who suffer from deafness. There is often a highly structured system of delusions and hallucinations, which may have a sexual content or which may relate to electrical appliances, for example. The response to antipsychotic drugs is good if concordance can be achieved. Newer agents, such as low-dose risperidone were thought to cause fewer long-term side-effects but increase the drug bill. As they have been used for longer it is also clear that they have a range of serious side-effects.

Depression

Prevalence

Depression occurs in around 10–15% of people aged over 65 years and is severe in 3%. The most important thing is to consider the possibility. If you are not sure, ask the patient – most will tell you and there is a surprisingly good correlation

---

'Graduate drinkers'

M=F
• Falls, confusion, gastrointestinal effects, self-neglect, anxiety, depression, hallucinations, Wernicke's encephalopathy, dementia, liver and heart complications.

'Late-onset drinkers'

F>M
• Attempt to assuage loneliness and sadness.
• Depression common.
• Complications similar to group 1.

Causes of hallucinations

• Paraphrenia.
• Poor vision (Charles Bonnett syndrome).
• Bereavement.
• Depression.
• Acute brain syndrome (including drugs, e.g. dopaminergic treatment for Parkinson's disease).
• Dementia.

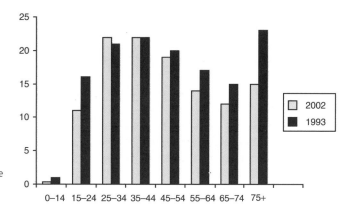

Figure 4.1 Mortality rates from suicide for men per 100,000 population (England and Wales).

between a yes/no answer to that question and a full psychiatric assessment. For an intermediate approach, screening tools such as the Geriatric Depression Scale (15-point version) may be helpful. Many old, ill people in hospital are anxious, lose their appetite, can't sleep or concentrate. In the list of features that follows, physical aspects are least helpful and anhedonia, perhaps the most.

Features

• Association with physical illness. Most chronic illness is associated with depression. Growing evidence suggests that there may be a subtype of depression in later life, characterized by a distinct clinical presentation and an association with cerebrovascular disease.
• Somatization of symptoms, hypochondriasis.
• Pervasive anhedonia ('when did you last enjoy anything?').
• Guilt, worthlessness, low self-esteem.
• Hopelessness and helplessness.
• Apathy or agitation, anxiety, delusions.
• Sleep disturbance.
• Withdrawal, poor concentration and memory ('pseudodementia').
• Self-neglect, malnutrition, dehydration.
• Suicide risk.

In almost all industrialized countries, men aged 75 years and older used to have the highest suicide rates. Suicide attempts in older people are often long planned, involve high-lethality methods and, as the elderly are more fragile and frequently live

alone, often lead to fatal outcome. In later life, in both sexes, major depression is the most common diagnosis in those who attempt or complete suicide. In England and Wales, the greatest reductions in male suicide rates have been seen in men over 75 years, from 26 per 100,000 population in 1989 to 15 per 100,000 population in 2002, suggesting that recognition and treatment of depression in old age has improved (Figure 4.1). However, a previous serious attempt, bereavement and isolation all point to high risk.

Treatment

Supportive

This involves counselling, relieving loneliness and practical measures, e.g. benefits check. Depression is often best managed with help of the local old age psychiatry service. In most areas this is a multi-professional group, with community psychiatric nurses (CPNs), social workers and a consultant. The team will carry out further assessment if necessary – usually in the patient's own home and will support them to continue with medication, etc. The old age psychiatry service may run a day hospital – many have different days for clients with depression or psychosis and dementia. Other options might include referral to Cruse Bereavement Care or arranging a day centre.

Sometimes the focus is on a patient, but the health needs of their carer are overlooked. Depression is extremely common amongst carers and it is essential to recognize this and offer support, such as arranging respite care or a sitting service such as Crossroads, before deterioration in the carer's mental health precipitates a crisis.

Drugs

SSRIs are the drugs of choice, having fewer sedating and anticholinergic effects than the tricyclic antidepressants and are relatively safe in overdose. Nausea, diarrhoea and restlessness can occur. To minimize nausea, start at a very low dose for the first week and gradually increase the dose. Give a simple explanation of the chemical basis of depression and explain that depression cannot just be shaken off by 'counting your blessings' or having a bit more moral fibre! Patients may have had bad experiences with benzodiazepines in the past, and so stress that these drugs are different, that they do not usually make them feel dopey but will need to be stopped gradually when no longer needed. Explain to the patient that any nausea will wear off and strongly reinforce the need to stick with the tablets for at least 6 weeks before expecting the cloud to lift. Information sheets can be useful. Treatment should be continued for a year or possibly even for life in severe cases.

There is no clear evidence that one SSRI is more efficacious or better tolerated by elderly patients than another. Other features may influence the choice of agent. For example, fluoxetine, fluvoxamine and paroxetine are more likely to be involved in significant drug–drug interactions than citalopram or sertraline. Everyone has their own favourites, but our current practice for most patients is citalopram starting with 10 mg. In special situations, the following are used: mirtazapine (a pre-synaptic α_2-antagonist, which increases noradrenergic and serotinergic transmission) where appetite stimulation is needed, trazadone (tricyclic with few antimuscarinic effects) if sedation is needed and venlafaxine (a serotonin and noradrenaline reuptake inhibitor) for resistant depression. If nausea is a major problem on SSRIs, lofepramine (a tricyclic with few antimuscarinic side-effects), building up from 70 mg may be helpful.

Electroconvulsive therapy

Electroconvulsive therapy (ECT) is comparatively quick and safe in severe cases but most psychiatrists are now very reluctant to consider ECT because of the bad press it has received. This is a great pity, as patients who were previously 'brought back' to a useful life now sometimes linger and die on their medication.

Dementia

Dementia, of which AD is the commonest cause, is a public health problem of enormous magnitude.

What is dementia?

Dementia is a *syndrome* (*lots of causes*) of *acquired* (*not learning difficulties*), *chronic* (*lasts months to years*), *global* (*not just memory or just language problems*) impairment of higher brain function, in an *alert patient* (*not drowsy*), which *interferes with the ability to cope* with daily living (it does not usually matter if an old person does not know 'it's Tuesday', but if he or she does not know 'it's winter', he or she might freeze).

Remember:

My (memory).
Old (orientation).
Grandmother (grasp).
Converses (communication).
Pretty (personality change).
Badly (behaviour disorder).

Source: From Brice Pitt, Emeritus Professor of Old Age Psychiatry at St Mary's, London.

Dementia contrasts with delirium, an acute confusional state with impaired consciousness. A person

---

Clinical features of acute confusion

- Onset typically abrupt.
- Marked fluctuation: lucid intervals.
- Altered consciousness.
- Inability to sustain, focus or shift attention.
- Disturbed cognition, e.g. disorganized thinking.
- Delusions and hallucinations.
- Fear, bewilderment, restlessness or hypoactivity.
- Possibly signs of underlying cause.

Causes of acute confusion

Intracranial
- Infarction – 'silent'; often frontal.
- Infection – meningoencephalitis.
- Injury – head injury, fat embolism.
- Iatrogenic – drugs acting on the CNS (including abrupt withdrawal, e.g. tranquillizers).

Extracranial
- Infection – especially chest, urine and cellulitis.
- Metabolic – fluid and electrolyte imbalance, hypoglycaemia, hypothermia.
- Anoxia – cardiac or respiratory failure, 'silent' myocardial infarction, carbon monoxide poisoning.
- Toxic – alcohol.
- Nutritional – Wernicke's encephalopathy.

can become delirious at any age, but frail older people often become confused when they are ill. An acute confusional state resolves as the underlying illness (e.g. chest or urinary infection) gets better. However, delirium is particularly common on a background of dementia, in which case the confusion will improve but only to a limited extent.

Treatment is summarized as follows:

1 Recognition: agitated delirium is usually obvious but apathetic delirium is easy to overlook.

2 Treat underlying cause.

3 Reassurance and explanation: avoid confrontation, use the family to sit with patient if willing.

4 Optimize environment and sensory input: glasses, hearing aid, dim light at night but avoid overstimulation.

5 Correct additional factors: fluid and electrolyte imbalance, nutritional deficiencies.

6 Avoid complications: low bed or mattress on floor to reduce risk of hip fracture, pressure mattress.

7 Restlessness, agitation: haloperidol, start with 0.5 mg, increasing if necessary in increments after 2 h; if neuroleptics are to be avoided, try lorazepam.

Causes of the dementia syndrome

The *primary dementias*, where the disease mainly affects the neurons in the brain, include AD, Dementia with Lewy bodies (DLB), other frontotemporal lobar atrophies including Pick's disease and frontotemporal dementia and Creutzfeldt–Jakob disease.

The commonest *secondary dementia,* in which the neuronal damage is secondary to pathology in other tissues, is vascular dementia (which includes multiple small infarcts and white matter ischaemia).

There is a rare familial form, CADASIL (cerebral autosomal dominant arteriopathy with subcortical infarcts and leucoencephalopathy), characterized by migraine, mid-adult cerebrovascular disease progressing to dementia and diffuse white matter lesions. Electron-dense granules in the media of arterioles can often be identified by electron microscopic evaluation of skin biopsies. More than 90% of the patients have mutations in the *Notch3* gene (chromosomal locus 19p). Molecular genetic testing is available.

Other important causes are drugs and alcohol, endocrine and metabolic problems such as thyroid dysfunction, recurrent or severe hypoglycaemia, post-hypoxia, nutritional problems such as vitamin B_{12} deficiency, brain tumours, trauma and infections including syphilis and HIV.

Remember:

Drugs and alcohol.

Eyes and ears.

Metabolic.

Emotional (really, psychiatric problems).

Nutritional.

Trauma and tumours.

Infections.

Atheroma – vascular dementia.

How common is dementia?

Dementia is rare below the age of 55 years but the prevalence of dementia increases dramatically with age to about *3% in the over 65 year olds* and rising to about *20% in the over 80 year olds*. There is a slight female preponderance. In elderly people, AD probably accounts for half to two-thirds of cases of dementia. About 800,000 people in the UK have dementia.

What happens in dementia?

The onset of dementia is insidious with gradual changes in memory and concentration, thinking processes, language use, personality, behaviour and orientation. Short-term memory is impaired early – long-term recall is often much better. Thinking becomes rigid and concrete. The condition progresses to obvious problems with short-term memory and managing basic activities of daily living, increasing disorientation and sometimes difficult or distressing behaviour such as night-time wandering, aggression or apathy. A tendency to lose things easily turns into paranoia and even delusions. Constant repetition of the same questions can be very trying for carers. Eventually, the patient is completely disorientated, no longer recognizes close family members, ceases to communicate and becomes doubly incontinent, bed-bound and totally dependent. Sadly, survival is often 8–10 years.

Why does dementia matter?

Dementia is a devastating condition for the patient while insight is preserved and for their family, who witness the progressive deterioration. For the spouse this has been likened to 'being bereaved without being widowed'. Dementia also has major economic consequences. Demographic changes are resulting in marked increases in the oldest old, one in five of whom may have dementia, a major cause of dependency and institutional care. Politicians and society are beginning to grapple with the issues and the cost of providing health and social care for patients with AD. In England, the direct costs of AD have been estimated at between £7.06 billion and £14.93 billion (2001), greater than the costs of stroke, heart disease and cancer. Long-term care for older people with cognitive impairment currently costs the UK £4.6 billion. By 2031 this is expected to rise by more than 130% to £10.9 billion. Unless treatments are found, the number of people with cognitive impairment who will be placed in institutions is expected to rise by more than 63% from 224,000 in 1998 to 365,000 in 2031.

In addition to the considerable morbidity, it is believed that AD is the seventh leading cause of death in the West. However, 'bronchopneumonia' usually appears on the death certificate. Despite this burden, dementia is only just beginning to command the attention it deserves.

How is a diagnosis of dementia made?

The GP is usually the first port of call, but a survey performed by the Alzheimer's Disease Society suggests that there is often difficulty in obtaining a diagnosis. Many old people are slightly forgetful and it can be difficult to distinguish ageing changes from early dementia. The term *age-associated memory impairment* is applied to a subjective complaint of forgetfulness in those over 50 years of age, with a performance on memory testing one standard deviation below the normal for a young adult. Almost 20% of people over 50 years of age meet these criteria and the significance is uncertain.

GPs may be reluctant to diagnose an 'untreatable' condition. If the patient lives alone there may be no one to give a history and unless a simple test of cognition is performed, it is easy to be misled by 'a good social front'. Quick screening tests include Hodkinson's Abbreviated Mental Test Score (see Appendix 4). However, if there are family members and they are concerned, there is usually a problem; whereas if only the patient is complaining, the diagnosis is often anxiety, depression or 'worried well'. Although dementia may have been developing for months, the patient often presents acutely because of a social crisis (e.g. death of caring spouse) or physical crisis (any illness, often a chest or urine infection, which worsens the confusion).

Having identified possible dementia, the GP may manage the patient or refer him or her to a geriatrician, an old age psychiatrist, a neurologist or, in some areas, a specialist memory clinic.

What are the aims of a clinical assessment?

Is it dementia?

A full history, with more detailed cognitive function testing, including assessment of language, visuospatial skills and reasoning (e.g. Mini-Mental State Examination (MMSE). Alzheimer's Disease Assessment Scale), usually answers this question. At this stage, other conditions must be ruled out.

The differential diagnosis includes an acute confusional state, depression, communication difficulties due to deafness, poor vision, or language deficits, PD, schizophrenia and mania.

Despite the lack of flexibility shown by NICE, it is important to understand that dementia does not equate with a number on a cognitive function score. Whether or not an individual presents with cognitive difficulties depends on their brain and the complexity of the environment in which they must function. A barrister with a European case brief may present with difficulty managing at work with an MMSE of 30, but a strong clinical suspicion confirmed by the passage of time that this is AD. An elderly resident in a care home who is described as not confused may have an MMSE of 16, as coping with the daily routine does not require a high degree of cognitive function.

What type of dementia is it?

The next step is to identify the cause. The dementia may be reversible (e.g. hypothyroidism), treatment may slow disease progression (e.g. treating hypertension in vascular dementia), specific treatment may be available (e.g. AD), genetic counselling may be required (e.g. familial AD) or it may be important to avoid certain medication (e.g. neuroleptics – also called antipsychotics or major tranquillizers – in DLB).

There is no diagnostic test for most of the primary dementias until a post-mortem examination,

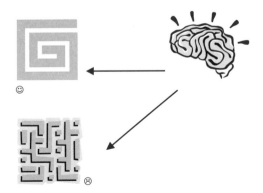

Figure 4.2 Presentation with dementia depends on the interaction between the brain and the environment.

so the *likely* cause is determined by the *clinical features* and the results of *investigations*. Common conditions such as vascular dementia and AD may co-exist and are probably additive.

Progressive deterioration is common in AD, whereas step-wise deterioration is characteristic of vascular dementia. Hallucinations and delusions are a feature of DLB. Parkinsonian features on examination would suggest vascular dementia or DLB. Most patients with dementia show some fluctuation, known as 'sundowning' because the confusion worsens in the evening, but this can be surprisingly marked in DLB. Weighted scores, such as the Hachinski ischaemia score, may improve diagnostic accuracy, and work is in progress to determine whether patterns of change found on neuropsychological and language testing add to diagnosis.

Investigations typically include blood tests to exclude reversible causes or other major pathology (blood count, biochemical profile, ESR, thyroid function, B_{12} and folate; syphilis serology and HIV testing are rarely relevant), CXR and ECG and a CT scan or MRI. In the late stages, a CT scan usually shows cerebral atrophy, but many patients with AD have a normal looking scan initially. The main purpose of the scan is to rule out a space-occupying lesion and identify major vascular disease. Genetic tests, such as determining the apolipoprotein E alleles that predispose to AD, are not routine.

Management

Management depends on the severity of the dementia, whether the patient lives alone and comprises a multi-disciplinary, multi-agency package of care. The package needs to be well coordinated and to evolve as the needs of the patient and carer change. Options include:
• Coping strategies and psychological techniques, reminiscence work and validation therapy.
• Optimize hearing, vision and improve general health.
• Treat other conditions which may impair cognition (e.g. anaemia, heart failure).
• Treat risk factors (e.g. hypertension in vascular dementia).

- Treat specific symptoms and behaviours (major tranquillizers, unfortunately, are often the only option).
- Education and support for carers (Alzheimer's Disease Society, Carers UK).
- Genetic counselling (only in rare early-onset dementias).
- Legal advice (e.g. a Lasting Power of Attorney may obviate the need for the Court of Protection at a later date, advice about driving, advance decisions, etc.).
- Therapy assessments (occupational therapy, speech and language therapy (for swallowing and communication) and physiotherapy; the aim is usually assessment to plan appropriate care and advise carers, rather than treat the patient).
- Assessment by social services (financial entitlements, especially attendance allowance, provision of services like home help and access to 'care management', the process by which frail old people are assessed for substantial packages of care at home or residential care).
- Regular district nurse/community psychiatric nurse support.
- Sitting services (Crossroads), day hospitals, respite care.
- Proper provision of long-term care.
- Palliative care in the terminal stages.

This list demonstrates just how much can be done in dementia. Until recently, drug management focused on the effects of the disease, e.g. major tranquillizers for disturbed behaviour. No drugs are licensed for the behavioural and psychological symptoms (BPSD) of patients with dementia. However, antipsychotics are widely used. Doses are lower than those in schizophrenia but Parkinsonian side-effects were common with first-generation drugs like haloperidol. The newer atypicals, e.g. risperidone, olanzapine, quetiapine, were seen as a step forwards, with fewer side-effects, but in a meta-analysis of 17 trials (modal duration of 10 weeks), the risk of death (variety of causes including cardiovascular) in drug-treated patients was 1.5 times that on placebo. In practice, once other measures have been tried, these drugs are still used. Use the lowest dose possible, and once the patient has settled, try to reduce and then stop the drug.

If possible explain the rationale and risks to the family.

Pathogenesis of Alzheimer's disease

Alzheimer's disease is divided into early-onset familial AD (EOFAD) and the usually sporadic late-onset form (i.e. LOAD). The pathology of both is identical with characteristic amyloid-containing extracellular plaques and the abnormal material which develops inside the neurons, the neurofibrillary tangles. In AD, amyloid beta-peptide (A), a fragment of a normal transmembrane protein, amyloid precursor protein, accumulates as plaques. According to the amyloid hypothesis, accumulation of A drives the pathogenesis of AD. The rest of the disease process, including formation of neurofibrillary tangles containing tau protein and cell death is proposed to result from an imbalance between A production and A clearance. The story is still developing – one new suggestion is that the memory loss is due to an abnormal form of the amyloid named A-beta star.

Three genes have been linked with EOFAD and all probably increase the brain levels of the amyloid precursor protein (see Table 4.1). LOAD also has a genetic component, the strength of which is debated, and is probably polygenic. The only definitely accepted association in LOAD is with apolipoprotein E4.

Risk factors for Alzheimer's disease

- Down's syndrome. Essentially all people with trisomy 21 develop the neuropathological hallmarks of AD after 40 years of age. More than half such individuals also show clinical evidence of cognitive decline. The presumed reason is the lifelong overexpression of the amyloid precursor protein and resultant over production of the A-amyloid.
- Age.
- Female sex.
- Apolipoprotein E4 genotype.
- Head injury.
- Elevated homocysteine levels (can be decreased by folate, so may be counterbalanced by fruit and vegetables in the diet).

Table 4.1 Genes associated with familial and sporadic AD – genes and Alzheimer's disease.

	Chromosome		
EOFAD			
β-amyloid	APP	21	Associated with Down's syndrome
Presenilin 1	PSEN1	14q	Commonest gene defect in EOFAD
Presenilin 2	PSEN2	1q	
LOAD			
Apolipoprotein E	ApoE	19q	Polymorphic: e2 e3 e4 are the common isoforms
			e4 is associated with atherosclerosis, coronary heart disease,
			vascular dementia, early onset AD and LOAD
?	10, 12		At least four other loci are postulated

Note: EOFAD, early-onset familial Alzheimer's disease; LOAD, late-onset Alzheimer's disease.

Protective factors for Alzheimer's disease

• Education (partly a threshold effect, but confounding with other associations with social class, e.g. diet high in antioxidants*).
• Continued brain activity (keep reading!).
• Tobacco (may be the nicotinic effect on cholinergic transmission, but not worth it).
• Wine and coffee (so it is not all bad news!).
• Exercise.
• Diet rich in foods containing vitamin E but not vitamin E supplements*.
• Non-steroidal anti-inflammatory drugs and aspirin. (observational – trials to date disappointing)
• Hormone replacement therapy (observational data supportive (fitter population) but not reproduced in trials.
• Treatment with a statin (could be reduction in vascular damage, evidence to date disappointing).

*Vitamin E supplements are not the same as the natural vitamin

---

A number of therapeutic approaches relating to amyloid are being developed – from small-scale trials of vaccines (one early study had severe side-effects in man) to Phase III trials of agents which alter aspects of amyloid biology, e.g. formation, deposition, metabolism and binding. IV Ig contains naturally occurring antibodies against A and is being tested, but is scarce and costly.

The metabolism of acetylcholine

(See fig 4.3.) The rationale for the drugs in current use for AD is earlier work showing that the brunt of neuronal death occurs in cholinergic projections. Cholinergic transmission could be enhanced by increasing the availability of the precursor, via direct stimulation of the receptors or by preventing the breakdown of endogenous acetylcholine. Three drugs, which are all acetylcholinesterase (AChE) inhibitors, are available:

• Donepezil – reversible inhibitor of AchE.

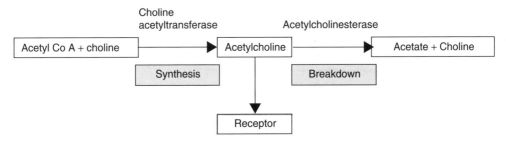

Figure 4.3 The metabolism of acetylcholine.

• Galantamine – reversible inhibitor of AChE with nicotinic receptor agonist properties.

• Rivastigmine – reversible non-competitive inhibitor of AChE and butyryl cholinesterase.

All have cholinergic side-effects especially nausea, vomiting and diarrhoea. To minimize these, the drugs are started at a low dose and gradually increased. Logically, with parasympathomimetic drugs (and with NSAIDs), care must be taken in sick sinus syndrome, peptic ulcer, COPD and urinary retention, and there may be interactions with muscle relaxants in anaesthesia. The drugs have limited efficacy and do not seem to benefit all patients, but many get a useful response in terms of memory or behaviour, with another 6 months of better function.

Acetylcholinesterase inhibitors are widely available in some countries but in the UK, there are restrictive guidelines (NICE, 2006):

• Diagnosis of AD made in a specialist clinic.
• MMSE 10–20.
• Carer's views considered and feasible to expect compliance.
• Drug continued if cognitive or behavioural benefit (stable MMSE indicates benefit as decline is expected).
• Six-monthly review and drug stopped if benefit no longer apparent or MMSE falls below 10.

Although the licensed indication is AD, trials have shown benefit in DLB and vascular dementia, and so the lack of diagnostic precision is not a danger. Although the cholinergic system is primarily affected, other neurotransmitter systems are involved and memantine, an N-methyl-D-aspartate receptor antagonist (which reduces glutamate-induced neurotoxicity) is licensed in the UK for the treatment of moderate to severe AD. It may be particularly useful for behavioural problems. However, NICE does not consider it cost-effective and recommends that it is only used as part of an ongoing trial.

In addition to anti-amyloid approaches and new cholinergic agents, ongoing drug trials in AD include statins, high-dose folate/B_6/B_{12} supplements, a combination of omega-3 fatty acids, uridine and choline (needed by neurons to make phospholipids) and lithium and valproate for agitation.

Dementia with Lewy bodies

Think of DLB if your patient seems to have a combination of symptoms of AD, PD, neuropsychiatric phenomena, particularly visual hallucinations and postural instability with wide fluctuations that can even involve conscious level. Lewy bodies, intracytoplasmic deposits of misfolded alpha-synuclein, are found throughout the cerebral cortex, whereas in PD they are restricted to the *substantia nigra*. DLB closely resembles the dementia typically associated with Parkinson's. Pragmatically, if cognitive symptoms precede physical symptoms by one year, the patient is considered to have DLB. Extreme care must be taken with all antipsychotic drugs as the patient may become drowsy, rigid and die.

Frontotemporal dementia

Frontotemporal dementia is characterized by gradual changes in personality, social behaviour, and language ability. Symptoms depend on whether the damage has primarily affected the right (behavioral problems) or left side (language deficits) of the frontal and anterior temporal lobes that control executive functioning. Frontotemporal dementia usually develops between 35 and 75 years of age and so, although it is rare (about 3% of dementia cases), it may present at an age when patients are labelled with AD. Orientation and memory are better preserved than in AD.

Pathologically, it is characterized by neurofibrillary tangles. These are known to be abnormally processed microtubule proteins. The microtubule-associated protein tau promotes tubulin polymerization and has a role in stabilizing the microtubules that are responsible for neuronal architecture and transport. A mutation in the *tau* gene causes a form of frontotemporal dementia called frontotemporal dementia with Parkinsonism linked to chromosome 17 (FTDP–17). Mutations in the *tau* gene impair the binding of tau protein to the microtubule and so frontotemporal dementia is one of the 'tauopathies'.

Transient global amnesia

This curious episodic disorder which predominantly affects older people is of unknown cause and is not predictive of stroke or dementia. In an episode the person remains alert and capable of high-level intellectual activity (e.g. driving), but if questioned may be perplexed and has impaired memory for past and present events.

Features

• Sudden-onset amnesia – retrograde for recent events, anterograde preventing new memories being laid down.
• Bemusement, perplexity, disorientation, repetitive questioning.
• Preservation of alertness, verbal fluency, motor activity.
• Duration a few hours, although complete recovery may take a few days; low recurrence rate.

Self-neglect

Old people are not infrequently encountered living in conditions of extreme degradation with total disregard for hygiene and self-care, the 'senile squalor syndrome'. Some will be found to have mental illness but others appear normal despite hoarding vast quantities of rubbish. This has been termed the Diogenes syndrome after Diogenes of Sinope, the ancient Greek philosopher who showed his contempt for material things by living in a barrel. He believed that happiness is attained by satisfying one's natural needs in the cheapest and easiest ways possible. In this context, the perpetrator is seen to have made a bizarre lifestyle choice, rather than having an illness, but the condition may lead to hypothermia, malnutrition and infections as well as vigorous protests from the neighbours!

Risk factors associated with self-neglect

• Dementia.
• Depression.
• Bereavement and isolation.
• Disability.
• Alcohol.
• Previous psychiatric disorder.
• Learning difficulties.
• Obsessive-compulsive disorder.
• Lifelong difficult personality/eccentricity.

Further information

Alcohol and the Elderly: www.ias.org.uk/factsheets/alcoholelderly.pdf

Alzheimer's Disease Education and Referral (ADEAR) Centre's National Institute of Aging website: http://www.nia.nih.gov/alzheimers

Alzheimer's Disease Society's website: http://www.alzheimers.org.uk/

Carers UK: http://www.carersuk.org/Home

Clinical trials in AD: http://www.clinicaltrials.gov/ct/action/GetStudy NIH website lists >120 trials in progress

Gatz, M., Reynolds, C.A., Fratiglioni, L., Johansson, B., Mortimer, J.A., Berg, S. *et al.* (2006) Role of genes and environments for explaining Alzheimer disease. *Archives of General Psychiatry*, **63**, 168–74.

Jacobsen, J.S., Reinhart P. and Pangalos M.N. (2005) *NeuroRx*, October; **2**(4), 612–26. Current concepts in therapeutic strategies targeting cognitive decline and disease modification in Alzheimer's Disease. Free full text on-line: http://www.pubmedcentral.nih.gov/articlerender.fcgi?tool=pubmed&pubmedid=16489369

Kelly, K.M., Nadon, N.L., Morrison, J.H., Thibault. O., Barnes, C.A. and Blalock EM. (2006) The neurobiology of aging. *Epilepsy Research*, **68**(Suppl. 1), S5–20.

Lewy body dementia website: http://www.lewybody.org/Home_Page.php

Mind – information on suicide: http://www.mind.org.uk/Information/Factsheets/Suicide/

NICE guidelines (2006): Donepezil, galantamine, rivastigmine (review) and memantine for the treatment of AD. Technology appraisal number 111. http://www.nice.org.uk/guidance/TA111/guidance/pdf/English.

Royal College of Psychiatrists Information on older people's mental health: http://www.rcpsych. ac.uk/mentalhealthinformation/olderpeople. aspx

Sorensen, S., Duberstein, P., Gill, D. and Pinquart, M. (2006) Dementia care: mental health effects, intervention strategies, and clinical implications. *Lancet Neurology,* **5**(11), 961–73.

O'Brien, J.T. (2006) Vascular cognitive impairment *American Journal of Geriatric Psychiatry*, **14**(9), 724–33.

Schneider, L.S., Dagerman, K.S. and Insel, P. (2005) Risk of death with atypical antipsychotic drug treatment for dementia: meta-analysis of randomized placebo-controlled trials. *JAMA,* **294,** 1934–43.

Chapter 5

Falls and immobility

Introduction

- Falls are *common:* one-third of over 65 year olds and one-half of over 80 year olds living in the community fall per year: and 50% of these are multiple falls.
- Women fall more frequently than men.
- Older people in nursing homes fall most often of all, because of their increasing frailty.
- Falls are *multi-factorial,* i.e. caused by the interplay between internal and external risk factors.
- Falls are not an inevitable part of ageing.
- Falls have important sequelae.
- Falls are a symptom, not a diagnosis.
- The National Service Framework for Older People Standard 6 addresses assessment and prevention of falls and osteoporosis.
- There are multiple guidelines available such as the NICE guidelines and RCP guidelines; see references at the end of the chapter.

Causes of falls

Most falls arise as a combination of internal factors, including gait and balance problems, medical, psychiatric and drug-related causes, and external causes, usually environmental.

A simple mnemonic for falls

DAME (reminds you that they are most common in women):
- Drugs (do not forget alcohol).
- Age-related changes (gait, balance problems and muscle weakness plus sensory impairment).
- Medical (cardiovascular disease, heart disease, Parkinson's disease (PD)).
- Environmental (obstacles, lighting, etc.).

Internal risk factors

Effects of ageing

- Body sway increases with age.
- Women have more body sway than men at any age.
- Reaction time slows down.
- Reflexes may be reduced.
- Walking patterns become less efficient and more irregular: worse with unsuitable footwear and neurological disease.

Medical causes of falls

Impaired sensory input
- Visual impairment (cataracts, glaucoma and inappropriate or dirty glasses) makes detection of

hazards difficult and dark adaptation is much slower, increasing the risk of falls at night.

- Impaired hearing and balance including vertigo and dizziness.
- Peripheral neuropathy makes walking difficult and potentially dangerous.

Drug-related

- Sedatives such as benzodiazepines and opiates impair insight and balance.
- Postural hypotension is often iatrogenic, e.g. diuretics for dependent oedema, treatment of PD.
- Cardiac arrhythmias may be iatrogenic, e.g. secondary to tricyclic antidepressants.
- Extrapyramidal side-effects secondary to neuroleptic medications.
- Polypharmacy, i.e. being on four or more medications correlates strongly with the risk of falling.
- Excess alcohol.

Gait abnormalities

- PD: the patient has difficulty getting going, the gait is shuffling and there is retropulsion.
- Hemiplegic gait: steps are slower, shorter and the gait is less smooth because the affected leg swings out in an arc.
- Cerebellar disease: a wide-base unsteady gait.
- Sensory ataxia: patient obviously watching the ground and their feet rather than looking ahead.
- Normal pressure hydrocephalus: again a wide-base ataxic gait.
- Antalgic gait: asymmetrical because the patient puts their weight on the side with the painful joint for as short a time as possible.
- Proximal myopathy: secondary to steroids and osteomalacia, e.g., produces a waddling gait.
- 'Scissoring' gait: osteoarthritis of the hips severely reduces the range of flexion at the pelvis during walking.
- Foot drop: high-stepping, foot-slapping gait, e.g. secondary to a common peroneal nerve palsy caused by a lower leg plaster cast fitting too tightly.

Reduced cerebral perfusion

- Cardiac – rate and rhythm changes and inability to maintain steady BP (see Chapter 9).

- Cerebrovascular transient brain stem ischaemia (see Chapter 7).
- Syncope: carotid sinus hypersensitivity, aortic stenosis or situational syncope, secondary to cough, micturition, etc. (see Chapter 9).

Epilepsy

The history is suggestive if there was a prodrome, e.g. smell of burning in temporal lobe epilepsy, longer duration of LOC with tonic clonic movements and cyanosis, incontinence and slow recovery associated with confusion and drowsiness (see Chapter 8).

Dizziness and unsteadiness

These are all descriptions of vague (heart-sink) symptoms. There are many possible causes, but they can be simplified into:

- Vascular disease which may respond to aspirin.
- Clinical cervical spondylosis, which may improve if a neck collar is worn.
- Review and stop any implicated medications including diuretics and advise to reduce alcohol intake if appropriate.

Psychiatric problems

- Dementia, especially Lewy body dementia, see the box below
- Delirium.
- Depression.
- Psychiatric medications, including antipsychotic medications and antidepressants.

External risk factors

- Older people tend to live in older housing, which may need repairs.

Risk factors for falls associated with dementia

- Loss of insight.
- Visuospatial problems.
- Extrapyramidal side-effects of antipsychotic medications.
- Drowsiness secondary to sedatives/antipsychotic medications.

- Poor lighting, especially near stairs.
- A lifetime's clutter.
- Inappropriate footwear such as slippers.
- Incorrect use of walking aids.
- Pets underfoot.
- Trailing electrical cables.
- Unfamiliar environment, e.g. hospital or a care home.

Sequelae of falls

Physical injuries

These occur in about one-half of reported falls.
- Soft-tissue bruising may require analgesics if mobility is to be maintained. Trauma may be reflected in raised muscle enzyme levels.
- Breaks in skin may be very slow to heal and grafting may be required.
- Fractures: orthopaedic treatment may be required in about 6% of falls.
- Friction burns from synthetic carpet when attempting to get up.
- Falls on to a fire or a hot surface, e.g. radiator, may result in a burn.
- Central-cord lesion leading to quadriplegia in patients with spinal cord compromised by spondylosis.

Psychological injury

- Fear of falling (Table 5.3) is increasingly being recognised as a common and important consequence of falls with significant effects on the future well-being of older people.
- Loss of confidence and mobility may result in older people becoming housebound or in need of residential care.
- Anxiety/depression about the future.

Social injury

- Because of intolerable anxiety in carers (formal and informal).
- Increased demands on carer may cause antagonism.
- The need to move to safer surroundings may separate faller from current supporters.

Death

- As a direct consequence of the fall.
- Up to 25% of frequent fallers are dead within 1 year of presentation, not directly due to injuries but because of underlying cause of falls.

Sequelae of a long lie

That is, remaining on the floor for 1 h or more after falling.
- Pressure sores (see Chapter 15).
- Hypothermia may result if fall occurs in the cold, e.g. outside or in an unheated room (see Chapter 12).
- Hypostatic pneumonia.
- Fifty per cent of those who lie on the floor for 1 h or more are dead within 6 months, even if no injury was sustained from the fall.

Determining the causes of falls

It is essential to get a witness report of the event surrounding the fall because:
- The patient may play down the event for fear of consequences.
- The patient may not remember blacking out, especially if the event was transitory.
- The witness can give information about the length of time of a blackout and whether there was associated tonic-clonic movements, and so on.
- The patient may have cognitive impairment.
- Research shows that even cognitively intact older people living in the community do not remember the falls after 3 months.

Aid to remembering what to ask: SPLATT!

- **S**ymptoms occurring: dizziness, chest pain, light-headedness, palpitations?
- **P**revious falls: is this the first fall secondary to an acute event or recurrent falls secondary to frailty/failing/dementia?
- **L**ocation: falls occurring outdoors have a better prognosis than those occurring in the home.
- **A**ctivity: walking, hanging out washing, extending neck, standing on chair?
- **T**ime: first thing in the morning whilst getting off the bed, after taking tablets, after a meal, and so forth?
- **T**rauma sustained?

Examination

Must be complete and thorough but pay particular attention to the following:
- Check the pulse rate and rhythm: massage the carotid sinus with ECG monitoring. See Chapter 9 for method and contraindications.
- Measure the BP – lying and after standing for 3 min. The drop is significant if it is more than 10 mmHg diastolic or 20 mmHg systolic and accompanied by symptoms. See Chapter 9.
- Look for sources of emboli – listen for murmurs, carotid bruits.
- Assess the CNS and look for lateralizng signs.
- Is there evidence of PD?
- Does the patient have myxoedema?
- Is there evidence of a peripheral neuropathy?
- Proximal myopathy: does the patient have difficulty getting out of the chair?
- Assess vision and hearing.
- Examine the neck movements. Does this cause dizziness?
- If the patient describes true vertigo, do the Hallpike manoeuvre.
- Assess the Mental Test Score.
- Baseline tests
- Full blood count (FBC)
- Thyroid stimulating hormone (TSH)
- Electrocardiogram (ECG)

Further investigations

The majority of falls are caused by problems with gait and balance. If falls continue and remain unexplained then it may be appropriate to investigate more aggressively:
- Holter monitor may show evidence of arrhythmia (the current thinking is that 48 h tapes have a greater yield than 24 h tapes, but there is no additional benefit from longer than this).
- Echocardiography will reveal aortic stenosis.
- Tilt table: measuring beat-to-beat variation in pulse and BP with the patient tilted to 70°. See Chapter 9 for further discussion.
- CT scan if multi-infarct disease suspected.
- If fits are the suspected cause, EEG and CT scan in selected cases need to be performed.

Treatment

The best way of approaching the management of falls is from a multi-disciplinary and multi-agency angle. Many hospitals now offer a Falls Prevention Clinic.
- Identify and treat *all* contributing causes and risk factors.
- Refer for physiotherapy. The aims are:
  (a) Correct prescription and use of walking aids. For example, people with PD often do better with wheeled frames to avoid the disruption to the flow of movements caused by having to lift the frame up.
  (b) Improve gait pattern, e.g. encourage people with PD to take longer steps.
  (c) Teach the patient how to get up from the floor.
  (d) Current evidence shows that individually tailored exercise plans do prevent future falls.
- Refer for occupational therapy assessment to identify and remove environmental hazards and provide equipment to facilitate mobility at home, and consider moving downstairs or getting a stair-lift.
- Challenge the need for all medication. Stop those that are unnecessary and try more patient-friendly alternatives where possible.
- Give advice on appropriate footwear: low heel for good heel strike but the soles should not be so thick that sensation is lost.

If no obvious causes are found, reduce the risks arising from the falls:
- Think about prevention of osteoporosis with calcium and vitamin D or bisphosphonates.
- Maintain a constant environmental temperature.
- Soften floor coverings, i.e. carpet rooms.
- Remove obstacles and dangers, e.g. guard fire.
- Place emergency bedding where it can be reached from the floor.
- Arrange for a personally worn alarm system or for frequent visitors.
- Teach the patient how to get up from the floor without help.
- Educate the patient and their relatives about safety in the home and the risk of falls: RoSPA

(Royal Society for the Prevention of Accidents) and Age Concern produce very helpful leaflets.

Hip protectors

- These are pads made from the same material as motorcycle helmets and work by diffusing the impact of a fall away from the neck of femur.
- They are worn over the greater trochanter and are incorporated in tight-fitting underpants.
- Community dwelling patients need to have good standing balance so that they can get the pants on and off.
- Because they are difficult to get on and off quickly, they may cause incontinence.
- The current evidence base has failed to show a decrease in the incidence of hip fractures.
- However, they may have a role in motivated community dwelling older people who understand the use of the hip protectors.

Falls in hospital

- Are very common.
- Are associated with cognitive impairment and acute delirium.
- May be due to unfamiliar surroundings and may be exacerbated by disturbed sleep and change in daily routines.
- May result in soft-tissue injuries and fractures.
- Prevention is under-researched.
- Understandably, relatives are often upset when a patient falls in hospital, as it is supposed to be a place of safety.
- The risk of falls can be reduced, but evidence suggests that patients should be allowed to optimize

their mobility and therefore some risk of falls has to be accepted.

- Always look for causes of delirium: especially chest infections, *Clostridium difficile*, UTIs, but also constipation.
- Review the medications, suspect opiates, benzodiazepines and all drugs that cross the blood–brain barrier. Do not forget, the patient may be receiving diuretics daily which they tend to omit at home and are therefore hypotensive.
- Try to maintain a calm environment. Frequently re-orientate the patient.
- Consider using a low bed, so that if the patient rolls out of bed, they will do themselves less harm.
- Remember that bed rails may reduce the risk of an obtunded patient rolling out of bed, but will do more harm if an agitated patient tries to climb over them.

Immobility

There are degrees of reduced mobility, ranging from not being able to drive, to being housebound and to being wheelchair-dependent. Immobility increases with increasing age. Over half of over 75 year olds have difficulty getting around their own homes. Among the ambulant aged 80 years, and over at least 25% will need some mechanical support when walking, such as a stick or frame. Generally, walking speed is reduced, with shorter, broader-based gait and increased time spent in 'double support', i.e. both feet in contact with the floor. Twenty per cent are totally housebound. Many older people find it difficult to climb on to a bus, and if they do manage it, there are other pitfalls: getting up from the seat, walking down the

Table 5.1 Immobility caused by pain/stiffness.

In joints	In muscles	In bones
Osteoarthritis	Myositis	Osteoporosis
Rheumatoid arthritis	Polymyalgia rheumatica	Osteomalacia
Gout	Myxoedema	Paget's disease
Pseudogout	PD	Malignant disease
Infection		

Table 5.2 Immobility caused by weakness.

Neuronal damage	Muscle damage	Reduced effort tolerance
Hemiplegia	Disuse	Dyspnoea
Peripheral neuropathy	Myopathy	Anaemia
Motor-neuron disease	Amyotrophy	Reduced cardiac output
Paraplegia	Hypokalaemia	

Table 5.3 Psychological causes of immobility.

Fear and anxiety	Re. falling
Manipulative behaviour	Attention seeking
Depression	Apathy reduces initiative
Dementia	Reduces insight into need to maintain mobility

crowded aisle possibly whilst the bus is still in motion and getting off at the correct stop. This coincides with the time that people are no longer able to drive because of failing vision, syncope, etc. (see Chapter 16).

Reasons for immobility

1 Pain and stiffness in bones, joints and muscles (Table 5.1). This is the most common reason.
2 Weakness, e.g. neurological or endocrine (see Table 5.2), but also generalized systemic disease.
3 Visual impairment and blindness.
4 Breathlessness secondary to pulmonary and cardiac disease.
5 Psychological problems: fear/anxiety/depression/dementia (see Table 5.3).
6 Frequent falls and fear of falling.
7 Iatrogenic, e.g. sedation, surgery (amputations and unsuccessful orthopaedic procedures).
8 Foot-care disorders, e.g. bunions and nail neglect; also severe ischaemia and infection.

Management of Immobility

• Ensure that there are no ongoing medical problems that are reversible.
• Refer fit patients with severe OA of the hips or knees for joint replacement.

Complications of immobility

Physical

• Muscle wasting (see Chapter 6).
• Osteoporosis (see Chapter 6).
• Muscle contractures.
• Pressure sores (see Chapter 15).
• Hypothermia (see Chapter 12).
• Hypostatic pneumonia.
• Constipation.
• Incontinence.
• Deep-venous Thrombosis (DVT) (see Chapter 9).

Psychological

• Depression.
• Loss of confidence.

Social

• Isolation.
• Risk of institutionalization.

• Optimize analgesia for patients with painful joints and backs.
• Review medication to ensure patient is not over-sedated, or has become Parkinsonian secondary to psychotropic medication or prochlorperazine.
• Refer to physiotherapy for review of posture, gait practice and use of correct walking aids. See Table 5.4.
• Check seat height correct for patient.

Table 5.4 Use of walking aids.

Walking aid	Description	Use	Disadvantages
Stick	Wood or aluminium. Correct length essential for functional gait pattern. Can be used singly or in pairs. Fisher grip: moulded hand grip may improve function.	Widens base of support and supports up to 25% of body weight. Use on same side for generally improving balance. Use on opposite side for painful/unstable joint.	Has to be propped up/laid flat when not being used and becomes a trip hazard! Check ferrules have not become worn.
Tripod/quadropod	Aluminium with three or four feet.	Gives more support than a stick and stands up on its own. The wider the base of the device, the wider the base of support. Used on opposite side of hemiplegia.	Can be large and ungainly.
Elbow crutches	Aluminium crutches with forearm support. Used in pairs.	Can support 80% of body weight. Useful for non-weight-bearing on a lower limb, e.g. because of amputation, or fracture.	Risk of tripping as above. Patient needs to have enough cognitive function to use them safely.
Axillary crutches	Crutches which bear the weight under the arms.	More often used for younger patients. Can achieve speed greater than normal walking!	Brachial nerve palsy if used too much.
Zimmer frame	Aluminium tubing with four rubber feet	Offers maximum support to patient. Bag or seat may be attached.	Patient has to be able to learn new gait pattern: the frame is lifted up and forward, and the patient then steps into the frame. This can be especially difficult on carpet. Encourages poor posture.
Rollator	As above, but there are wheels on the two front legs	Patient can push the frame continuously; especially useful for patients with PD.	Poor posture, slow gait, problems walking outdoors
Gutter frame	Has support for the forearms	Useful for patients with rheumatoid affecting their wrists, and wrist injuries	As above
Delta frame	Usually a three-wheeled foldaway frame, often with a seat/space for shopping	More robust so can be used outside	Heavy

• Ask podiatrist to help with painful in-growing toe nails, onychogryphosis, bunions, and so on.

• If the patient is likely to remain immobile, ensure that they are assessed for pressure relieving equipment on the bed and chair. Monitor skin condition and nutrition. See Chapter 15.

Further information

Age Concern website: www.ageconcern.org.uk

Guidelines for the Prevention of Falls in Older Persons (2001) *Journal of American Geriatrics Society*, **49**, 664–72.

Home and Leisure Accident Research (1988) *Accidents and Elderly People.* Department of Trade and Industry, London.

Lord, S.R., Sherrington, C. and Menz, H.B. (2001) *Falls in Older People: Risk Factors and Strategies for Prevention.* Cambridge University Press, Cambridge.

National Patient Safety Age slips, tips +falls in hospital www.npsa.nhs.uk/site/media/documents 2350-0488-PSO-falls-summary-WEB.pdf

NICE Guidelines on Falls: www.nice.org.uk pdf CG021NICEguidelinepdf

Royal College of Physicians: Falls and bone health: www.replondon.ac.uk/college/ceen/fbhop/.

Royal Society for the Prevention of Accidents website: www.rospa.co.uk

Studenski, S. (1996) *Clinics in Geriatric Medicine – Gait and Balance Disorders.* W.B. Saunders, Philadelphia, PA.

Wynne-Horley, D. (1991) *Living Dangerously: Risk Taking, Safety and Older People.* Centre for Policy on Ageing, London.

Chapter 6

Bones, muscles and joints

Bones

Ageing changes

Bone structure changes throughout life owing to ongoing bone resorption by osteoclasts and bone growth by osteoblasts. With increasing age, the balance is lost, leading to increased bone resorption. This in turn leads to gradual and progressive loss of bone from the age of 35 onwards. This process affects trabecular bone more than cortical bone. The bone histology is normal, but the total bone mass is markedly reduced.

Bone loss per year is 0.2% of the total from the age of 35 and increases to 1% after the menopause in women. This means that, on average, by the age of 80, a woman will have lost 30% of her bone mass whilst a man of the same age will have lost 10%.

The shape of long bones changes with increasing age; the internal cavity increases in diameter, the outer cortical layer becomes thinner and the total bone diameter becomes expanded. These changes result in weaker bones.

Osteoporosis

Risk factors for osteoporosis

- Age >60.
- Female sex.
- Family history of osteoporosis, especially maternal hip fracture.
- Failure to maximize bone density in adolescence and early adulthood because of poor nutrition or oestrogen deficits, e.g. secondary to anorexia nervosa.
- Hormonal changes at the menopause: the fall in oestrogen causes acceleration of bone loss. Fractures secondary to osteoporosis affect one in two post-menopausal women.
- Previous fragility fractures.
- Low body weight.
- Physical inactivity.
- Use of corticosteroids for 3 or more months.
- Other drugs especially caffeine, antiepileptics, alcohol and cigarettes.
- Endocrine disorders, e.g. thyrotoxicosis, Cushing's disease, hyperparathyroidism and hypopituitarism.
- Falls are not a cause of osteoporosis, but are strongly predictive of osteoporotic fractures.
- Older people often have vitamin D deficiency and secondary hyperparathyroidism, and these are likely to contribute.

Osteoporosis in men

- Affects 20% of men over 70 years of age.
- One in five men over the age of 50 will sustain a fracture.
- Fifty per cent of men affected have idiopathic osteoporosis.
- In the other 50%, the most common causes are:
  - Hypogonadotrophic hypogonadism.
  - Steroids.
  - Alcohol.
  - Hyperparathyroidism.
  - Malabsorption, e.g. secondary to Crohns' disease, gastric surgery and coeliac disease.

- The reduction of insulin-like growth factor production is also being investigated as a risk factor.

Clinical features

Osteoporosis is usually asymptomatic until there has been a fracture:

- Often the first presentation is a Colles' wrist fracture in women aged 50–65 years old.
- Vertebral fractures may present as severe mid-thoracic or low back pain often with no history of trauma.
- Loss of height and dorsal kyphosis secondary to multiple vertebral fractures. A loss of >4 cm suggests at least one vertebral fracture.
- Contact between ribs and iliac crests.
- Hip fractures: rising incidence with increasing age. The incidence is rising faster than expected from demographic changes. There are now 57,000 cases per annum in the UK – 75% of which are aged over 75.
- Other fractures associated with osteoporosis include neck of humerus, pelvis and distal tibia/fibula.

Fractured neck of femur

- Increasingly common in the ageing population.
- The number predicted worldwide in 2050 is 6.26 million.
- Presents as pain in the hip with inability to weight bear, although if it is an impacted fracture, the patient may still be able to walk.
- The affected leg is shortened because the hip is flexed and externally rotated.
- The fracture is surgically fixed according to its site.
- The timing of the operation is controversial. The best compromise is as soon as reasonably possible when patient's medical condition is optimized.
- The patient does best if mobilized early.
- The reasons for the fall should be sought and treated if possible.
- National Institute for Health and Clinical Exellence (NICE) guidelines suggest that women over the age of 75 who sustain a fracture should be commenced on treatment for osteoporosis.
- Twenty per cent of patients have died within 1 year of the fracture.
- Twenty per cent require institutional care.

Fractured pelvis

- Usually the pubic rami. Remember that the pelvis is a ring and is therefore likely to fracture in two places.
- Often caused by trivial trauma.
- Produces pain in the groin that is worse on walking and getting up from sitting.
- Treatment is conservative with analgesia and early mobilization.
- Most heal within 6–8 weeks.

Investigations

Bone mineral density The dual-energy X-ray absorptiometry (DEXA) scanner measures bone density usually at the proximal femur and lumbar vertebrae. Osteoporosis is defined as a bone mineral density (BMD) of greater than 2.5 standard deviations (SDs) below that of a normal pre-menopausal woman and is expressed as a T score (i.e. T–2.5 SD).

Ultrasound of the calcaneum This has the advantage of being inexpensive and portable so that it can be used in the primary-care setting but has not been fully validated. It is probably most useful at risk stratification, and so if the result suggests low bone density, the patient should have DEXA scan.

Excluding causes of secondary osteoporosis If serum calcium is raised, check PTH level to exclude primary hyperparathyroidism (see section on Primary hyper-parathyroidism in this chapter).

- TFT: (thyroid function tests) to exclude thyrotoxicosis (see Chapter 12).
- Testosterone: in men with suspected hypogonadotrophic hypogonadism.
- ESR and serum immunoglobulins to exclude myeloma.
- Dexamethasone suppression test to exclude Cushing's disease.

Complications of osteoporosis

- Fractures, as earlier.
- Deformity: kyphosis, loss of height, abdominal protrusion. Cord compression is very uncommon.
- Loss of independence and risk of being admitted to a care home.
- Use of resources: 25% of UK orthopaedic beds are occupied by patients with fractured hips. The average cost is £25,000 per patient. Fractures in osteoporotic bones now account for over 1 million

bed-days annually in the National Health Service (NHS). The cost of treatment of these patients is now more than £5 million per week.

Prevention

- Adequate nutrition.
- Calcium and vitamin D.
- Hormone replacement therapy is most useful in women in early menopause.
- Exercise: should be regular and weight-bearing, e.g. walking.
- Prophylactic use of bisphosphonates: if treatment with steroids, dose greater than 7.5 mg of prednisolone for 3 or more months.

Treatments

1 Calcium and vitamin D. It has been shown that treatment with calcium and vitamin D prevents hip fractures in older people living in care homes. There is controversy about role in other populations; research is ongoing. All the trials looking at the efficacy of bisphosphonates, strontium and teriparatide have co-prescribed calcium and vitamin D preparations.

2 Bisphosphonates, e.g. risedronate and alendronate, work by binding to hydroxyapatite in the bone, thus inhibiting bone resorption. Effects are seen in the first 12–18 months of use. Both are shown to increase bone mass of the spine and the hip and to reduce fractures. Weekly and monthly preparations are now available. This is an advantage because bisphosphonates are taken on an empty stomach to ensure absorption. Thus, patients only miss their early morning cup of tea once a week! The patient also has to remain upright for 30 min to reduce the risk of oesophageal ulceration. Side-effects include gastric irritation, abdominal pain, diarrhoea and constipation. Bisphosphonates are effective in the biologically younger population.

3 Strontium ranelate is said to increase bone growth and reduce bone loss. It comes in a sachet to be mixed with water and usually is taken at bedtime. It is an alternative for those who do not tolerate the bisphosphonates.

4 Teriparatide is recombinant PTH, which is given once daily by subcutaneous injection for 18 months. Given intermittently, it is anabolic,

contrary to the effect of endogenous PTH, and is useful in severe osteoporosis, where it is believed that bisphosphonates will be insufficient. Its use is restricted to metabolic bone specialists because it is expensive.

5 Selective oestrogen modulators (SERMs), e.g. raloxifene, act as oestrogen agonists in the bone and liver but as oestrogen antagonists in the breast and uterus, and therefore increase bone density without increasing the risk of breast or uterine cancer.

6 Calcitonin can be given as an intramuscular injection, and is a useful adjunct in pain control following an acute wedge fracture.

7 Analgesia is essential for all osteoporotic fractures.

8 Treat causes of secondary osteoporosis.

9 Internal fixation of NOF.

10 Balloon kyphoplasty is a promising new treatment for vertebral collapse, as it restores the vertebral body height, reduces pain rapidly and thus enables patient to mobilize.

Prevention of further fractures

- Treatment of osteoporosis.
- Exercise programmes.
- Falls prevention strategies (see Chapter 5).
- The use of hip protector pads is controversial (see Chapter 5).

Osteomalacia

This is reduced calcification of the osteoid matrix due to vitamin D deficiency. The amount of bone is normal, but it is soft and weak compared with normal bone.

Incidence

Is uncertain and depends on population studied:

- Admissions to Scottish departments of geriatric medicine, 4%.
- Post-mortem study of elderly patients, 12%.
- Biopsies on fractured neck of femur patients, 25%.

Causes

Reduced vitamin D availability

- Deficient diet.

• Reduced sun exposure: most common in Muslim and Hindu cultures (where women wear headgear that shields them from the sun) and in institutionalized elderly people. Sunlight is essential for 1-hydroxylation of vitamin D.

• Malabsorption, e.g. secondary to coeliac disease, diverticular disease of the small bowel and postgastrectomy.

Impaired vitamin D metabolism

• Chronic renal failure (the kidney is the site for 25 hydroxylation of vitamin D).

• Drugs that induce liver enzymes, e.g. phenytoin and carbamazepine.

Clinical features

• Pain in the axial skeleton (spine, shoulders, ribs and pelvis).

• Muscle weakness.

• Waddling gait and difficulty standing from sitting secondary to osteomalacic myopathy.

• Fragility fractures.

Investigations

• X-rays may show insufficiency fractures, Looser's zones.

• Bone scintigram may show 'hungry bones', so-called because the bones take up the isotope so readily that they are very bright and the kidneys may not be visible.

• Blood tests: raised alkaline phosphatase, low corrected calcium and low phosphate.

• Serum 25 hydroxyvitamin D_3 will also be low.

• Bone biopsy will clinch the diagnosis where there is doubt.

Treatment

• Oral vitamin supplements, e.g. vitamin D and calcium.

• In the case of abnormal metabolism, e.g. renal disease, give 25 hydroxylated preparation, alphcalcidol or calcitriol.

• Watch for hypercalcaemia.

Paget's disease of the bone

This is a localized abnormality of bone that arises because of increased activity of the osteoclasts and osteoblasts. The net result is an increase in bone turnover, which produces bone that is increased in size, but is paradoxically weaker than normal bone. Paget's disease of the bone most frequently affects the pelvis, spine, skull and the femur, although any bone can be affected. A single bone is affected in 10% of cases. The adjacent bone may also be affected.

Incidence

The incidence increases with age. The prevalence is 5% of over 40 year olds, rising to 10% of over 90 year olds.

Aetiology

This is still unknown, but there is likely to be a link between environmental and genetic factors. There have been studies linking it to parvovirus. A candidate gene has been found on chromosome 18q2. There is also a link with HLA DQW 1 antigen.

Clinical features

• It is usually asymptomatic and is diagnosed incidentally on X-rays.

• Pain, localized or secondary to nerve entrapment.

• Deformity, e.g. enlargement of the skull, anterior bowing of the tibia or lateral bowing of the femur.

Investigations

1 Raised serum alkaline phosphatase.
2 Raised urinary hydroxyproline suggest active disease.
3 Serum calcium is raised in patients who are immobile.
4 X-rays show the bones to be enlarged, abnormally dense and distorted.

Complications

- Fractures of abnormal bone.
- Secondary osteoarthritis of adjacent joints.
- Neurological: compression of the cranial nerves as they exit the skull, most commonly affects the eighth nerve, but can also affect the second and the fifth; or paraplegia if the spinal cord is compressed.
- Hydrocephalus.
- High-output heart failure caused by Paget's disease of the bone is very rare.
- The development of malignant tumours is also rare, but examples include osteosarcoma, and chondrosarcoma.

Treatment

- Aimed at treating pain and preventing deformities and fractures.
- Acute disease is treated with a bisphosphonate, usually risedronate, which reduces disease activity (mirrored by a fall in serum alkaline phosphatase and urinary hydroxyproline) and pain within days of starting treatment.
- Risedronate is usually given for 2–6 months.
- Treatment can be repeated if necessary.
- Intravenous pamidronate can be given if an oral preparation is not tolerated or if the disease is rapidly progressing.

Primary hyperparathyroidism

Incidence

- Two-hundred fifty-five cases per million per year.
- Occurs worldwide.
- Fifty-five per cent of cases will be women over 70 years of age.

Clinical features

- The majority of elderly patients will be asymptomatic and the problem will have been discovered on biochemical testing done for other reasons.
- Asymptomatic patients should simply be observed and their biochemistry monitored.

- However, 12% of cases with a raised calcium level will have had documented episodes of confusion and dehydration and will merit treatment if otherwise well.
- Check PTH level.
- Sesta MIBI scan: technetium 99 is preferentially taken up by overactive parathyroid glands to demonstrate the anatomy prior to surgery.
- Minimally invasive parathyroidectomy is now available, with good results and short hospital stays.

Hypercalcaemia

There are many causes of hypercalcaemia. In practice, the following are the main groups affecting older people:
- Primary hyperparathyroidism, as mentioned earlier.
- The hypercalcaemia of malignancy may be due to bone metastases but also non-metastatic manifestation of malignant disease.
- Myeloma (see Chapter 14).
- Drug induced: thiazide diuretics, lithium and vitamin D.
- Renal failure (see Chapter 13).
- Sarcoidosis, hyperthyroidism and Addison's disease are rare causes in this age group.

Emergency treatment involves rehydration with intravenous normal saline plus loop diuretics if there is fluid overload. Intravenous pamidronate is an effective treatment especially in malignancy.

Joints

Many people accept joint problems as a part of growing older – but arthritis is not universal, and in old age it must be as precisely diagnosed as possible so that appropriate treatment and management may be instigated (Table 6.1).

Osteoarthritis

- Osteoarthritis (OA) is the most common joint disorder and the incidence increases with increasing age.

Table 6.1 Patient consulting rate per 1000 persons (by age in years) for patients with joint diseases.

	Joint diseases: consulting rate				
All ages	0–14	15–44	45–64	65–74	75
34	2	14	62	105	114

- Three-quarters of people over the age of 65 years have some X-ray evidence of OA.
- Two-thirds of people over the age of 65 years have symptoms from OA.
- Small changes in management may produce big improvements in quality of life and symptom control.
- Joint abnormalities arise because of failure of normal repair of cartilage and periarticular bone after injury, leading to damage of the cartilage and abnormal new bone formation, such as osteophytes and secondary changes in the synovium.
- Long-standing, complicated and burnt-out rheumatoid arthritis may be difficult to differentiate from generalized OA in old age.
- Aetiology usually unknown, i.e. primary osteoarthritis.
- May be secondary to:
  - Genetic predisposition.
  - Repetitive heavy loading of the joints.
  - Obesity.
  - Trauma leading to articular deformity.
  - Inflammatory disease, including gout and rheumatoid arthritis.
  - Aseptic necrosis.
  - Endocrine disease, e.g. myxoedema and acromegaly.
  - Neuropathic, e.g. diabetic, and therefore painless.
  - Hereditary disease, e.g. haemophilia.
  - Metabolic disease, e.g. Wilson's disease, haemochromatosis, homocysteinuria.

Symptoms

- Pain: gradual in onset, intermittent, worse on movement and relieved by rest.
- Sleep may be disturbed in severe cases.

- Joints most often affected are DIPs, PIPs, base of thumb (painless but unsightly), hips, knees and cervical and lumbar spine.
- Hip pain is worse in the anterior groin and may radiate into the buttock or thigh.
- Knee pain worse in the anterior knee and patellofemoral joint, but may be referred to the hip.
- Early morning stiffness should last no longer than 15 mins.
- Functional problems include difficulty bending down to put on shoes, getting out of a chair and walking long distances, which eventually may lead to immobility.

Signs

- Tenderness and bony swelling secondary to osteophytes and swelling due to effusion.
- Painful, reduced range of movement.
- In OA of the hip, the leg may be shortened because the hip is flexed and externally rotated and there may be marked quadriceps wasting.
- Crepitus.
- Eventually the joint may become deformed, e.g. genu valgus (knock knees) and varus (bow knees), bunion.
- Gait may be antalgic, i.e. less time is spent with weight on the affected side.

Treatment

Pharmacological
- Simple analgesia, such as paracetamol taken regularly can be enough to control pain.
- NSAIDs should be reserved for flare-ups because of multiple side-effects. COX-2 inhibitors, such as rofecoxib and celecoxib, are designed to preferentially treat inflammation without causing GI symptoms.

However, they have been associated with increased risk of thrombotic heart disease.

- Capsaicin is derived from chilli peppers and applied topically can give good pain relief.
- Intra-articular steroid injection can produce pain relief for a period of 2 weeks, sufficient to allow a patient to enjoy a special occasion, but is not indicated for long-term treatment.

Non-pharmacological

- Weight loss relieves the strain on the joints.
- Physiotherapy is aimed at improving the range of movement, strengthening muscles surrounding the joint and thus stabilizing the joint.
- Using a stick in the opposite hand or a frame can reduce the load on an affected hip or knee by 50%.
- Hot and cold packs for temporary relief of pain.
- Joint replacement.

Complications of joint replacement

- Infection: affects about 1% of hip replacements. Usually prophylactic antibiotics are given. The most common infection is a simple wound infection. A deeper infection may be more difficult to diagnose; a gallium scan can be helpful.
- DVT: subcutaneous low-molecular-weight heparin is usually given as prophylaxis.
- Loosening of prosthesis: X-ray or bone scan may demonstrate this.
- Fracture of adjacent bone: visible on X-ray.
- Patient outlives prosthesis and second operation needed.

The ideal patient for joint replacement

- Refractory pain in single joint or only one severely affected joint.
- Physically fit.
- Well motivated.
- Mentally alert and orientated.
- Well nourished, but not obese.
- Unlikely to place unreasonable demands on new hip, i.e. normal mobility anticipated post-operatively and not excessive activity.
- Of sufficient age so that patient is unlikely to outlive the new joint. About one-quarter of replacement hips need revision after 10 years.

- Increased mobility reveals an additional pathology, e.g. angina results from the increased activity.

Rheumatoid arthritis (RA)

The incidence is about 1% worldwide in older people.

- *Inactive disease* An episode in earlier life which has burnt itself out but leaving many deformities and disabilities, sometimes progressing to a mixture of old rheumatoid arthritis and more recent osteoarthritis. The treatment is the same as for osteoarthritis.
- *New disease* Arising in old age for the first time can be difficult to differentiate from polymyalgia rheumatica.
- Exacerbation of old disease.

Active rheumatoid disease

- May have very sudden and severe onset in old age.
- May be self-limiting.
- Equal sex incidence (females no longer predominate).
- Fewer systemic complications.
- Treatment may be more hazardous in old age.

Potential problems in the treatment of rheumatoid arthritis in elderly patients

Splinting of joints If bulky and heavy, may significantly interfere with frail person's ability to maintain personal independence. Night splints are more acceptable to some patients.

Rehabilitation The presence of severe upper-limb problems and other disorders will significantly hinder a patient's ability to cooperate fully in an intensive physiotherapy programme.

Drugs These are often dangerous in old age, but important and valuable:

1 Quick symptom relief may be the best way to preserve mobility and independence; therefore steroids (in spite of disadvantages) may be used earlier than in younger patients.

2 Disease-modifying anti-rheumatic drugs (DMARDs) may act too slowly to benefit older people. Also, there is increased risk of side-effects

because of age and pathological changes in other systems, e.g. renal impairment worsened by penicillamine and gold and visual impairment potentiated by chloroquine. The role of the anti-tumour necrosis factor agents, such as infliximab, has not been assessed in the older population.

3 The mainstay of treatment in active disease is with NSAIDs, but all complications of treatment are more pronounced in the elderly.

4 It was hoped that COX-2 inhibitors would inhibit synovial prostaglandins without inhibiting intestinal prostaglandins thus relatively sparing the GI tract. Unfortunately, their use has been associated with an increased risk of thrombotic cardiovascular events.

Crystal arthropathy

Recurrent episodes of sudden severe pain causing immobility are often due to an acute inflammatory response to either urate (gout) or calcium crystal (pseudogout) deposition in a joint. All causes are age related and sex incidence in old age approaches equality. See Table 6.2 for a comparison between the two types.

Note that both gout and pseudogout may be confused with acute joint sepsis. Aspiration for pus and crystals is the best technique for differentiation.

Infective arthropathy

• Should be considered when a single joint is painful.
• Difficult to diagnose in presence of old joint deformities.
• May be confused with gout or pseudogout.
• Systemic toxic effects may be minimal in the elderly.
• Concurrent treatment may mask the problem, e.g. steroids, analgesics and antibiotics.
• Aspirate if in doubt.

Table 6.2 Clinical features, precipitating factors and treatment of crystal arthropathies.

	Gout	Pseudogout
Type of crystal	Urate	Pyrophosphate
Appearance under polarized light	Negatively birefringent	Positively birefringent
Joints most commonly affected	MTP joint of great toe, ankle, PIP joints of fingers,	Large joints, most commonly knee
Precipitating factors	Diuretics, overindulgence, fasting, uric acid containing foods such as strawberries, acute illness or surgery, blood malignancies	No acute precipitant may be identified, but acute illness or surgery often responsible
Extra-articular features	Tophi may be present around the affected joint, or on the pinna	None
Serum uric acid	May be raised or normal in an acute attack	Normal
X-ray appearance	Erosions	Linear opacification of articular cartilage
Treatment of acute episode	NSAIDs, colchicine, steroids, rest	NSAIDs, rest
Prevention	Allopurinol	None
Associated conditions	Obesity, hypertension, IHD	Diabetes, myxoedema, hyperparathyroidism
Family history	Common	Less common

Muscle pain

Polymyalgia rheumatica

Generalized muscle pain and tenderness. Probably due to an arteritis and linked with giant-cell arteritis – usually idiopathic, but may be triggered by a viral infection or may indicate the presence of an underlying malignancy.

Epidemiology

- Most common in people aged 60–70.
- Male to female ratio is 2:1.
- Incidence is 20/100,000 per annum.
- It is the most common reason for commencing older people on steroids.

Diagnostic criteria

1 Bilateral shoulder pain and/or neck stiffness.
2 Onset of illness of less than 2 weeks.
3 Initial ESR greater than 40.
4 Duration of morning stiffness of more than 1hr.
5 Age greater than 65 years.
6 Depression and/or weight loss.
7 Bilateral tenderness in upper arms.

Three positives are suggestive of polymyalgia rheumatica. Those features higher in the list are most strongly predictive of polymyalgia rheumatica. A successful therapeutic trial with steroids will confirm diagnosis: the response is often dramatic.

Note: Creatinine phosphokinase, muscle biopsy and EMG are all usually normal.

Complications of untreated polymyalgia rheumatica

- Chronic disability.
- Normochromic anaemia.
- Hepatitis with raised alkaline phosphatase.
- The patient may become immobile.
- Progression to giant-cell arteritis with major-vessel occlusion, leading to blindness, stroke or myocardial infarction.

Treatment

1 Steroids: 20 mg prednisolone daily is sufficient for polymyalgia rheumatica. Higher doses are necessary if giant-cell arteritis is suspected (see Chapter 9). Rapid improvement in symptoms helps to confirm the diagnosis.
2 Dosage should be monitored according to symptoms and elevation of ESR.
3 Bone protection should be given. Use calcium and vitamin D in older, frailer people and bisphosphonates in biologically fitter people.
4 Treatment may be necessary for 2 years or more and disease may recur and require a further course of steroids.
5 NSAIDs may help to resolve symptoms of PMR, but will not protect the patient from vascular occlusion.

Muscle weakness

Ageing changes

Muscle bulk and effectiveness decline with increasing age. Muscles become atrophic and paler in colour due to a decrease in the number of muscle fibres, an increase in fat and fibrous tissue and increased deposition of lipochrome pigment. These changes are not exclusively due to ageing, but merely reflect the more sedentary life in old age in developed countries. Muscle bulk can still be increased in old age by regular exercise. Neuronal impairment may be another explanation for the 'ageing changes'.

Muscle pathology in old age

Myositis

- Tender and weak muscles.
- Serum creatine phosphokinase usually elevated.
- Rarely infective in old age, but transient post viral symptoms are common.
- Often associated with underlying malignancy.
- Often associated with skin involvement – dermatomyositis: patchy red/ purple rash often on knuckles/ eyelids.

Myopathy

- Weak muscles usually proximal and without tenderness.
- Non-metastatic complication of malignancy commonest cause.
- Endocrine – Cushing's; thyrotoxicosis; diabetic amyotrophy.
- Drug-induced, e.g. statins, steroids and alcohol.
- Metabolic, usually due to hypokalaemia (endocrine or drug induced).
- Also vitamin D deficiency (part of osteomalacia).

Myasthenia gravis

- Exaggerated fatigue, e.g. of the eye muscles causing ptosis or diplopia.
- Ten per cent of all cases occur in older age.
- The majority in this age group are idiopathic.
- Diagnosis is by correction of the symptom with use of the short acting anticholinesterase edrophonium chloride (Tensilon® test). There may also be autoantibodies to antiacetylcholine receptors.
- May be associated with underlying malignancy, in which case the response to Tensilon® is poor.
- May be drug induced (penicillamine and aminoglycosides).

Investigation of muscle disease

1 Raised creatine phosphokinase indicates muscle damage.
2 An EMG helps differentiate neurogenic and primary muscle disorders.
3 Biopsy – difficult and requires skilled and experienced interpretation; therefore best results from specialized centres.

4 Tensilon® test – in suspected myasthenia.
5 Specific tests to confirm underlying cause, e.g. thyroid-function tests.

Treatment

- Correct precipitating cause, if possible.
- Anticholinesterases in myasthenia, e.g. pyridostigmine.
- Steroids are worth trying in malignant myopathy, especially polymyositis/ dermatomyositis, but beware of causing steroid myopathy.

Further information

DTi Report 2000: *The Economic Cost of Hip Fracture in the UK*.http://www.dti.gov.uk/files/file21463.pdf.

Guidelines Working Group for the Bone and Tooth Society, National Osteoporosis Society and Royal College of Physicians. Glucocorticoid induced osteoporosis: guidelines for prevention and treatment. Website: www.rcplondon.ac.uk/pubs/books/glucocorticoid/index.asp.

Hamerman, D. (ed.) (1988) *Clinics in Geriatric Medicine – Rheumatic Disorders*. W.B. Saunders, Philadelphia, PA.

Misbah, S.A. (ed.) (2001) *Rheumatology and Clinical Immunology*. In: *Medical Masterclass* (Firth, J.D. editor in chief). Blackwell Science, Oxford.

Poole, K.E.S. and Compston, J.E. (2007) Osteoporosis and its management. *British Medical Journal*, 333, 1251–56.

SIGN Guidelines for Management of Osteoporosis; www.sign.ac.uk/guidelines/fulltext/71/index.html

Chapter 7

Stroke made simple

Importance

Anyone can have a stroke, including babies and children, but the vast majority – n i n e out of ten – affect people aged over 55. Each year over 150,000 people in UK have a stroke. Stroke is the third most common cause of death, after heart disease and cancer (11% of all deaths). Stroke is the largest single cause of severe disability in developed countries and is very expensive as patients need prolonged rehabilitation and, sometimes, care for life. A quarter of a million people in the UK are living with long-term disability as a result of stroke. Managing stroke in a stroke unit (multi-disciplinary, coordinated care) produces marked benefit. For every 16 stroke patients admitted to a general ward, there would be one more death than in a stroke unit.

Definition

A stroke or cerebrovascular accident (CVA) is defined as 'rapidly developing clinical signs of focal (or global) disturbance of cerebral function, with symptoms lasting 24 h or longer or leading to death, with no apparent cause other than of vascular origin'. This includes subarachnoid haemorrhage (SAH) but excludes subdural haematoma and haemorrhage into a tumour. By definition, a transient ischaemic attack (TIA) lasts less than 24 h, and so TIAs are classified separately, but the causes of TIA and stroke are very similar. TIAs are a risk factor for stroke.

Outcome of stroke

The outcome of a stroke (Table 7.1) depends on the volume and part of brain that is affected, the fitness of the patient and co-existing conditions. You will see a range of figures for outcome, depending on the population in the study, but overall the rule of thirds is useful: one-third die (most within the first 10 days), one-third make a good recovery within a month and one-third suffer residual impairment, disability and handicap (about one-half moderate, and one-half severe).

Aetiology and pathology

A stroke results from interruption to the brain's blood supply due to an infarct or a haemorrhage. An infarct is an area of ischaemia (usually due to thrombosis *in situ* or an embolus from the carotids or heart but occasionally due to low BP from any cause or damage to the blood vessel wall).

Table 7.1 Outcome of stroke.

1-month mortality	25–50%
1-year mortality of survivors	40%
Full or almost full recovery	25–50%
Return to work if previously working	30–35%
Unable to walk outdoors	40%
Unable to walk unaided	20–25%
Long-term high-dependency care	12–20%

A primary haemorrhage may be due to an arterial abnormality, such as an aneurysm, but both infarcts and bleeds usually occur in vessels damaged by hypertension and atheroma. Sometimes there is secondary bleeding into an area of brain damaged by an infarct. The proportions of the types of stroke vary in different countries: in the UK atherothrombotic strokes comprise 80% and in Japan haemorrhagic strokes are much more common. The biggest risk factor for stroke is increasing age, but it is more useful to consider risk factors that can be treated.

Risk factors for stroke are similar to those for other vascular disease such as ischaemic heart disease (IHD) and peripheral vascular disease (Table 7.2). However, there are differences in relative risk that are not understood, e.g. smoking is a bigger risk for IHD and hypertension is a bigger risk for stroke. In future, there may be increased understanding of the role of inflammation as high CRP (though still within the 'normal range') is emerging as a risk factor for vascular disease. In general, primary and secondary risk factors are similar. Risk factors tend to multiply. As there is more chance of another vascular event once one has occurred, the risk–benefit ratio for treatments changes. (This is why healthy 40-year olds are advised not to take aspirin as their chance of a bleed outweighs likely benefits).

Presentation

Typically, the onset is abrupt. Occasionally a hemiparesis develops over a period of 12 or more hours but, if it progresses over days or a week or two, a space-occupying lesion (SOL), such as a tumour or subdural haematoma, should be suspected. Other conditions that may mimic stroke are hypoglycaemia and Todd's (post-epileptic) paresis.

A stroke may present as coma of unknown cause, in which case neurological examination requiring cooperation is impossible. Stroke presents with coma in three situations:
1 Brain stem infarct.
2 Large cortical infarct with brain stem compression.
3 Seizure after stroke.

In a brain stem stroke, signs are often bilateral and the pupils may be small. In a major cortical stroke, the cheek on the paralysed side may flap in and out with respiration and the limbs on that side are likely to have completely lost all tone. Reflexes may be unhelpful at this stage. One finding that, if present, pretty well wraps up the diagnosis is conjugate deviation of gaze towards the side of the lesion, due to the unopposed effect of the contralateral frontal eye field (remember, the patient 'looks away' from a tumour but towards a stroke). Loss of consciousness points towards a severe stroke, but by no means inevitably towards cerebral haemorrhage as the pathology.

The conscious or slightly drowsy patient usually presents little diagnostic difficulty. The peak time of onset for stroke is in the early hours of the morning and, if capable of speech, the patient will describe waking up and trying to get out of bed, only to find him or herself unable to walk. An eyewitness may relate that in the middle of a meal the patient dropped his or her cup and developed facial asymmetry and difficulty with speech and then became unable to stand or perhaps even sit properly. Examination will then usually reveal characteristic deficits: in the early stages, the paralysed limbs are more often flaccid than spastic and in some cases they stay that way. Establish the exact time of onset (unfortunately impossible if the patient woke from sleep). If it is less than 3 h, act fast as thrombolysis may be possible (see subsequent text).

Clinical types of stroke

Transient ischaemic attacks

These are isolated or recurrent focal neurological symptoms (usually negative) attributed to platelet emboli from an atheromatous plaque or ulcer in the aorta, the common carotid artery or, most often, the carotid bifurcation or red-cell emboli from the heart. Monocular loss of vision (amaurosis fugax) hemi- or monoparesis, dysphasia and unilateral sensory disturbance are examples within the internal carotid territory. The problem must resolve within 24 h to be called a TIA, but most last

Table 7.2 Primary and secondary risk factors.

Risk factor	Management	Goal
BP high	Promote healthy lifestyle; diet (see below), moderate alcohol intake and exercise. Treat BP if still high with drugs individualized to patient (e.g. age, race, need for drugs with specific benefits), but ACE inhibitor/ diuretic combinations may have a particular role	<140/85 mm/Hg; <130/85 mm/ Hg if renal insufficiency or heart failure; <130/80mm/ Hg if diabetic
Heart disease	As appropriate for the condition, also aiming to reduce platelet stickiness, minimize LVH and maintain in sinus rhythm	Reduce chances of embolization
Atrial fibrillation	Verify AF on ECG or paroxysmal AF on 24 h tape. For patients in chronic or inter-mittent AF, use warfarin aiming for INR 2.0–3.0 (target 2.5). Aspirin is used if there are contra indications to oral anticoagulation. Low-risk patients <65 years may be treated with aspirin	Anti-platelet drugs if 'low risk' but anticoagulation for PAF or AF.
Sticky platelets	Aspirin (75–300 mg) except in intolerance and brain haemorrhage, caution with asthma and history of GI haemorrhage, with modified release dipyridamole (ESPRIT study) for 2 years after vascular event. Clopidogrel if aspirin intolerant.	Concordance with long-term anti-platelet therapy
Carotid stenosis	Anti-platelet therapy, document degree of stenosis and offer endarterectomy if CT confirms stroke in ipsilateral hemisphere, function worth preserving and stenosis >70% or >50% if over 75 years	Ensure eligible patients with anterior circulation strokes are screened: the fit elderly have most to gain
Smoking	Check smoking status, advise quitting and refer for support, e.g. clinic/pharmacological help (nicotine or buproprion)	Quit and avoid passive smoking
Unhealthy diet	Advocate low-fat, low-salt, high fruit and vegetable diet with weight loss if needed. Discourage excess consumption of any food, however 'healthy', to avoid health scares, e.g. heavy metals in oily fish	Varied healthy diet

(Continued p. 66)

Table 7.2 Continued

Risk factor	Management	Goal
Obesity	Calorie restriction and increased caloric expenditure	Achieve and maintain desirable weight (BMI 18–25 kg/m2). Higher BMI is less of a risk if central obesity is not present
Excess alcohol	Low/moderate alcohol intake protects from atherothrombotic stroke (amount probably depends on individual as increase in BP and obesity may be adverse) but high or binge intake is a risk for haemorrhage	Avoid binge or excessive drinking
Adverse lipid profile	Give advice about diet, weight and exercise but unless total cholesterol <3.5 start simvastatin 40 mg. Refer to specialist if triglycerides/ total cholesterol remain high.	It is likely that the lower the total cholesterol, the better
Diabetes and impaired glucose tolerance	After diet and exercise, second-step therapy is usually oral hypoglycemic drugs: sulphonylureas and/or metformin with ancillary use of acarbose and thiazolidinediones. Then consider insulin.	Normal fasting plasma glucose (<7 mmol/L) and near normal HbA1c (<7%)
Lack of exercise	Medical check before initiating vigorous exercise programme: start slowly if older or unfit. Moderate-intensity activities (40–60% of maximum capacity) are equivalent to a brisk walk. Additional benefit from vigorous (>60% of maximum capacity) exercise for 20–40 min on 3–5 days/week	At least 30 min of moderate- intensity physical activity on most days of the week
Previous TIA	Treat all risk factors	

Notes: BMI, body mass index; GI, gastrointestinal.

less than a couple of hours, usually just a few minutes. The distinction between a TIA and a very small infarct is somewhat academic. The risk of stroke after a hemispheric TIA is up to 20% in the first month, highest in the first 72 h; so after a TIA, anti-platelet treatment should be started at once and the person referred to a rapid access TIA clinic. Doppler duplex imaging or magnetic resonance angiography is mandatory for subjects suitable for endarterectomy.

Transient ischaemic attacks also occur within the territory of the vertebrobasilar circulation, although true vertebrobasilar ischaemia or insufficiency is something of a diagnostic dustbin and is very rare. The main features are true vertigo (a sensation of rotary movement of either patient or surroundings), true drop attacks (sudden falls due to total loss of tone without disturbance of consciousness and with rapid and complete recovery) and diplopia, although cortical blindness, tetraparesis,

ataxia and dysphagia may also occur. Vertebrobasilar insufficiency does not require intervention other than aspirin. TIAs are not a cause of loss of consciousness.

The established stroke

Detailed descriptions of the enormous variety of syndromes explicable in terms of the precise anatomy of the damage sustained are beyond the scope of this book. The identification of the major deficits is more important and the classification devised by Bamford in 1991 (Table 7.3) is simple and provides useful prognostic information.

Clinical problems following stroke

Dysphagia Difficulty with swallowing is common initially (see Management of the established stroke, p. 69).

Table 7.3 Brain infarction.

	Clinical	Anatomy/ pathology	Outcome
TACI (15%)	Higher cerebral dysfunction (e.g. dysphasia, dyscalculia, visuospatial disorder) and hemianopia and ipsilateral motor and/or sensory deficit involving two out of three of face, arm or leg	MCA occluded by embolus/spreading thrombus from ICA	Very poor chance of good function and high mortality
PACI (35%)	2/3 TACI components or higher cerebral dysfunction alone or restricted motor/sensory deficit (e.g. one limb or face, hand, not whole arm)	Branch of MCA or ACA	Fair outcome but very high chance of early recurrence
LacI (25%)	Pure motor, pure sensory or sensorimotor or 'ataxic hemiparesis'	Lipohyalinosis of deep perforating artery	Often good recovery
PoCI (25%)	Cranial nerve palsy with contralateral motor/sensory deficit or bilateral motor/sensory deficits or dysconjugate eye movements or cerebellar deficit/hemianopia	Brain stem, cerebellum or occipital lobes	High chance of good function but also of recurrence in 1st year

Notes: ACA, anterior cerebral artery; ICA, internal carotid artery; LacI, lacunar infarct; MCA, middle cerebral artery; PACI, partial anterior circulatory infarct; PoCI, posterior circulatory infarct; TACI, total anterior circulatory infarct.

Source: Bamford (1991).

Dysphasia Disorder of language affecting some right-handed patients with left-hemisphere lesions:
• Anterior dysphasia – non-fluent, impaired naming.
• Posterior dysphasia – often fluent, jargon type, receptive dysphasia.

Fluent dysphasia is often confused with 'acute confusion'! In left-handers, two-thirds have left-sided speech dominance; those who have right-sided dominance may/may not develop dysphasia, irrespective of side of lesion.

Dysarthria Disorder of articulation in which the content of the speech is unaffected. This can be due to unilateral VII palsy but otherwise suggests bilateral disease (or pathology in the cerebellum or basal ganglia).

Dyspraxia Inability to perform purposeful movement despite adequate comprehension and motor function. Varieties include dressing apraxia.

Sensory neglect Visual – exclude hemianopia first. Test by line bisection, line cancellation (Albert's test). Tactile, if gross, includes loss of body image and denial of problem.

Visuospatial perception Non-dominant hemisphere lesion – besides tests includes asking the patient draw simple objects such as house, face, clock face.

Weakness of limbs Usually develop increased tone, marked 'clasp-knife' spasticity and flaccidity are both adverse.

Sensory loss Any modality, gross-position sense loss is highly adverse.

Hemianopia Major handicap unless patient aware and able to compensate by turning head.

Depression Especially in dominant-hemisphere lesion. Treat with antidepressants.

Thalamic pain Try antidepressant or anticonvulsant.

Shoulder pain Subluxation especially likely following traction on the weak arm.

Multi-infarct disease (dementia)

This condition is also known as 'lacunar state' and is seen in arteriopaths and those with atrial fibrillation (AF). The features are:
• History of hypertension.
• Step-wise progression.
• Neurological signs depending on location.
• Dementia when lacunae total 50–100 mL.
• Abnormal gait marche à petits pas, broad-based backward-leaning.
• Pseudobulbar palsy:
  (a) Dysarthria.
  (b) Dysphagia.
  (c) Emotional lability.

Cerebellar infarct or haematoma

Requires special mention because:
1 'Stroke somewhere–stroke nowhere = stroke in the cerebellum' (or, it should be added, thalamus, especially if there is a severe memory deficit).
2 Surgical evacuation to decompress the posterior fossa is often beneficial; biologically fit patients should be discussed with the neurosurgeons.

Spinal-cord infarction

This may cause sudden paraplegia or quadriplegia and is often caused by a compressing lesion. Spinal cord ischaemia can cause 'neurogenic claudication' and mimic peripheral vascular disease.

Subarachnoid haemorrhage

This should be considered if the patient presents with severe sudden-onset (thunderclap) headache with or without neurological signs. CT scan should be performed urgently if conscious level is impaired, or else within 12 h. If CT is negative, LP should be performed after 12 h to look for xanthochromia. If the diagnosis is confirmed, oral nimodipine 60 mg 4 hourly is started; supportive measures are similar for a stroke with codeine as analgesia. Discuss the patient urgently with a neurosurgeon. If the plan is active management, they will be transferred that day and the vasculature will be imaged. A ruptured aneurysm may be clipped or ablated. Treatable complications include secondary hydrocephalus. If there is a family history of SAH or polycystic renal disease, genetic counselling is needed. Long-term BP control must be strict.

Central venous thrombosis

This may present like a stroke, but there is often a history of headache and fits. It is rare but more common if there is a prothrombotic tendency, e.g. disseminated malignancy or sinus infection. The damage does not follow a typical arterial territory. MRI is often needed for diagnosis. Although there is often bleeding into the brain – treatment is with heparin.

Investigation of stroke

Typical tests may include: FBC, CRP, glucose, renal, liver and bone function, cardiac enzymes if concomitant MI is possible (troponin appears more cardio-specific than CK-MB), cholesterol and thyroid function, ECG, CXR, cardiac echocardiogram and 24 h tape if cardiogenic embolus is suspected, and carotid Doppler studies. ESR, CRP and autoantibodies may be useful in infection or if vasculitis is a possibility.

Brain CT scan is now standard, with the exception of patients who appear so likely to die so that any intervention seems unjustified. The area of low attenuation characteristic of an infarct often

---

Indications for CT for stroke patients
1 Suspicion of SOL.
2 Atypical presentation.
3 Head injury.
4 Known malignancy.
5 Suspicion of SAH.
6 Suspicion of meningitis.
7 Need to distinguish infarct from haemorrhage (most common indication as almost always determines treatment).
8 Possible cerebellar haematoma.

does not become apparent for 24 h, and techniques are being developed for early visualization. Haemorrhage is immediately apparent as a white area (Figure 7.1). MRI may help in small lesions, unusual situations and is better than CT for the brainstem and posterior fossa.

Management of the established stroke

Where?

Patients with minor stroke can be managed at home, provided there is sufficient family support and adequate community rehabilitation. Most, however, are admitted to hospital, mainly for nursing support. Whatever the setting, proper diagnosis (usually brain CT), identification of risk factors and initiation of measures for secondary prevention are essential. Even in the early phase, management of a stroke patient is multi-disciplinary.

If the patient is admitted to hospital, the outcome is much better if the patient is managed on a *stroke unit*. It is unclear which component of stroke unit care leads to the improved outcome, but stroke units have been the most important advancement in stroke in the last decade. Thereafter, rehabilitation can take place in the patient's own home, in a community hospital or in a day hospital, depending on circumstances.

General care

Blood glucose, arterial oxygen, hydration and temperature should be maintained within normal

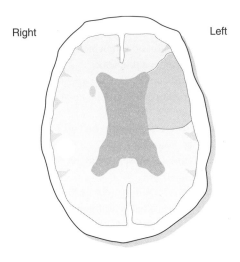

Figure 7.1 Diagram of head-CT showing appearances of a parietal haematoma and a deep lacunar infarct on the right and a TACI on the left.

limits. Complications, such as pressure sores and chest infection (consider aspiration), may be present on admission and are treated in the usual way. Prevention of further complications is essential. The unconscious patient will need full nursing care with particular attention to airway, pressure areas and bladder drainage. Thromboembolic device stockings (TEDS) may be beneficial in patients with reduced mobility (check foot pulses before prescribing). Although subcutaneous heparin reduces deaths from PE, haemorrhagic deaths are increased; so heparin is usually not used. Correct positioning and chest physiotherapy are needed. High BP is usually only treated acutely if it is likely to produce its own complications, e.g. hypertensive encephalopathy. Aspirin (300 mg) should be given as soon as primary haemorrhage is ruled out, and then 75 mg is given daily, via a nasogastric (NG) tube or rectally if the patient is dysphagic.

Dispersing the thrombus

Trials of thrombolysis have shown benefit in very selected patients when given soon after stroke onset. More patients suffer intracranial haemorrhage but overall fewer have severe disability at 3 months. Intravenous recombinant-tissue-type plasminogen (rt-PA) activator (alteplase) is approved by the US Food and Drug Administration and UK Medicines Agency for treating acute ischaemic stroke within 3 h of onset of symptoms. Post-marketing data suggest that the risk of intracranial haemorrhage may be unacceptably high when rt-PA is given to patients who would not have been eligible for enrolment in the clinical trials. Practical problems include getting patients to hospital, performing CT scan within the time frame and interpreting the early scans. Aspirin is delayed for 24 h after thrombolysis.

Vasodilatation and cerebral oedema

No convincing advantage has emerged from various trials of vasodilators, partly because the vessels in the infarcted zone are already maximally dilated. The same applies to various agents designed to relieve cerebral oedema. Trials of haemodilution have also been unsuccessful.

Neuroprotection

In a stroke there is a central zone of irreversibly damaged cells surrounded by a penumbra of ischaemic but potentially salvageable cells. These face a number of threats including oedema, the release of glutamate, aspartate and lactate and an influx of calcium ions. The penumbral tissue increases its oxygen extraction (normally about 40%) from the available blood for a day or two after the event, indicating the time scale available for intervention. Trials of N-methyl-D-aspartate (NMDA) receptor blockers, which prevent the released glutamate from causing a toxic influx of calcium ions into the neurons, have been disappointing. This may be an example of poor extrapolation from animal work to the clinical situation: glutamate does kill neurons immediately after brain injury, but preserves endangered neurons in the long term. The only way to provide neuroprotection with NMDA antagonists would be to administer them before the insult and for a very short period (minutes) after the injury, which is impossible in a stroke.

Hydration and nutrition

There are four situations in which taking fluid and nutrition becomes a problem:
1 The unconscious or drowsy patient (transient).
2 Pseudobulbar palsy due to bilateral stroke (often prolonged).
3 Brain stem stroke with bulbar involvement (sometimes prolonged).
4 The common hemisphere infarct (usually transient) (about 40%).
It is usual to put the patient on a nil-by-mouth regime until the patient's swallow has been assessed by the speech and language therapist or trained stroke nurse. Inadequate airway protection does not equate with an absent gag reflex, nor is the reverse true. The ability to swallow fluids is assessed by sitting the patient up and observing his or her ability to swallow a teaspoon (5 mL), a tablespoon (15 mL) and then 50–100 mL of water. Sensitivity

of this observation is improved by monitoring oxygen saturation during the procedure. If the patient is unable to swallow, pooling occurs in the mouth. Choking and obvious aspiration with coughing may ensue, but some patients aspirate 'silently', which is where monitoring the oxygen saturation is helpful. Fluid and electrolytes are given intravenously. One advantage of this route is that eventually the line 'tissues', which provides an opportunity to decide whether or not to resite it. In a patient who is clearly doing very badly, artificial hydration may not be relevant. Fluid (usually about a litre a day) may also be given subcutaneously.

Sooner or later the decision must be taken whether to feed as well as to hydrate the persistently dysphagic patient. The usual practice is to offer nutrition via a fine-bore NG tube at around 72 h after the stroke. The FOOD trial supported early NG tube feeding, but at the risk of increasing the proportion of survivors with poor outcome. It is rare for an NG tube to remain in place for more than a few days as they are easily dislodged. If the swallow still fails to recover, the NG tube may be 'bridled', which makes it difficult to dislodge, or a percutaneous endoscopic gastrostomy (PEG) tube may be considered usually at around 14 days but this procedure should not be undertaken lightly. Remember, the purpose of feeding tubes is to nourish and hydrate, not to protect the airway; they do not prevent aspiration of contaminated oral secretions or regurgitated gastric contents. This needs to be explained to many nurses as well as the family. Decisions about hydration and feeding are difficult ethically, particularly after a stroke. Always seek senior advice.

Information for the family or patient

Depending on the severity of the stroke the patient and or the family need appropriate information. Leaflets from a patient-based society such as the Stroke Association are very helpful.

If the patient is not doing well, the team should make a decision about whether to attempt cardiopulmonary resuscitation (CPR) in the event of cardio-respiratory arrest. This is a clinical decision based on the patient's condition. It may be possible to discuss this with the patient or find out from the family what they feel the patient would have wanted. In the context of a major stroke, CPR is most unlikely to be successful. If recovery is very poor, end-of-life decisions, such as the futility of repeated antibiotic treatment, should be discussed.

Rehabilitation

The first week of stabilization of the stroke is followed by 2–3 weeks of rapid recovery and then a further 6 months of slow but continuing improvement. Although the impairment may only achieve a further 10% of recovery during this phase, the resultant disabilities can often take longer and therefore show greater late improvement. The multi-disciplinary aspects of rehabilitation are discussed in Chapter 3.

The sequence of sitting, transferring, standing and walking may therefore take a couple of months if the hemiparesis is initially quite severe. In general, proximal movements recover better than distal and lower limbs more than upper. Visual problems may be helped by referral to an orthoptist. Prisms may be helpful for persistent diplopia and hemianopia and advice may be given about compensatory strategies. Depression is common after stroke, both initially and after discharge home when the elation at making it home is tempered with the reality of the residual handicap.

Primary and secondary prevention

This overlaps with prevention in IHD and is detailed Table 7.1.

Indicators of poor outcome

- Severity of stroke, e.g. TACI.
- Significant cognitive impairment.
- Admitted comatose.
- Persistent incontinence.
- Paralysis of conjugate gaze.
- Neglect, persistent visuospatial perceptual disorder.
- Homonomous hemianopia.
- Depression and other reasons for poor motivation.
- Significant associated pathology.
- No grip at 3 weeks – useful hand function unlikely.

Driving after a stroke

It is advisable for the patient to inform his or her insurance company in the event of stroke or TIA. Driving may be resumed after 1 month if there is no residual deficit; if there is a deficit, the Driver and Vehicle Licensing Authority (DVLA) must be informed and formal assessment may be required.

Information on discharge from hospital

Despite the fact that simple lifestyle changes like healthy eating, exercise and stopping smoking can significantly cut the risk of a second stroke, the Healthcare Commission (2005) found that nearly half of stroke patients were not given any information about dietary changes and a third were not given advice about physical exercise. The risk of a recurrent stroke is around 35% within 5 years. Even moderate physical activity can reduce the risk of stroke by up to 27% and eating five portions of fruit and vegetables a day can cut the risk of stroke by 25%. Patients also need full information about their medication, out-of-hospital services, equipment including assistive technology, benefits, carer's services and local support groups.

Further information

Bamford J., Sandercock P., Dennis M., Burn J. and Warlow C. (1991) Classification and natural history of clinically identifiable subtypes of cerebral infarction. *Lancet*, **337**, 1521–6.

Cochrane library website for regularly updated stroke reviews from the Cochrane library (search the Abstracts): http://www.update-software.com/cochrane/

Dennis, M.S., Lewis, S.C. and Warlow, C. (Food Trial Collaboration). (2005). Effect of timing and method of enteral tube feeding for dysphagic stroke patients (FOOD): a multicentre randomised controlled trial. *Lancet*, **365**, 764–72.

ESPRIT Study Group. (2006) Aspirin plus dipyridamole versus aspirin alone after cerebral ischaemia of arterial origin ESPRIT: randomised controlled trial. *Lancet,* **367**, 1665–73.

Ikonomidou, C. and Turski, L. (2002) Why did NMDA receptor antagonists fail clinical trials for stroke and traumatic brain injury? *Lancet Neurology*, **1**, 383.

Massachusetts medical students' website written with the American Stroke Association: http://www.umassmed.edu/strokestop

Royal College of Physicians National Clinical Guidelines for stroke second edition 2004 http://www.rcplondon.ac.uk/pubs/books/stroke/stroke_guidelines_2ed.pdf

Stroke association website: http://www.stroke.org.uk/

Washington University School of medicine website has a record of trials in progress so you can see which drugs may make a clinical impact shortly: http://www.strokecenter.org/trials/.

Young, J. and Forster, A. (2007) Review of stroke rehabilitation. *British Medical Journal*, **334**, 86–90.

Chapter 8

Other diseases of the nervous system

Age changes and clinical examination

A full examination of the CNS can be an ordeal for both a frail elderly patient and his or her doctor. Patience and understanding are required by both and compromise will often be needed.

Much can be gained by simply observing the patient. The patient's memory and speech during history taking and their ability to walk to and get on to the examination couch may give you clues to underlying pathology.

Ageing changes and co-morbidities, e.g. arthritis may confuse the clinical picture. Gait changes with age, becoming slower and less regular in pattern, with feet closer together, less firm heel strike and more time with both feet on the ground. The older the patient, the more difficult are the problems – almost one-third of 'normal over 80 year olds' walk with a shuffling gait and almost half have a flexed posture but most do not have PD.

Muscle wasting is common, usually in the proximal muscles, due to disuse; this is especially a problem in very elderly women, who may find it very difficult to rise from a chair without assistance. For this reason, chairs in out-patient clinics should have arms. Wasting of the small muscles, of the hand, does not automatically have the sinister connotations of the same finding in young subjects.

Reflexes may be difficult to elicit because of other pathologies, e.g. osteoarthritis and ankle jerks in particular are difficult to elicit in almost one-third of elderly people. Abdominal reflexes are almost universally absent.

Pupils are often small and react sluggishly and, for these reasons, plus cataracts, examination of the fundi is often difficult or impossible (even after mydriasis).

Fine changes in sensation may be difficult to determine – moving from abnormal to normal is generally easier for patients to detect. Vibration sense is often lost or not understood, so position sense is usually a better test to employ (but fixed joints may make even this difficult).

Do be gentle with your patients if you want their cooperation. If necessary, break the CNS examination down into stages and do not expect perfection from yourself or your patient.

Symptomatic classification of neurological disease in the elderly

1 Headache:
  • Raised intracranial pressure but fewer than 10% of patients with brain tumour present with headache alone.
  • Pain radiating from cervical spondylosis.
  • Giant-cell arteritis – superficial, with tender arteries, tenderness over proximal muscles, high ESR/CRP.
  • Psychological – but the prevalence of 'tension' headaches declines with age, consider depression.

- Paget's disease of the skull is occasionally painful when active – often obvious.
- Migraine but new-onset migraine is unusual over 50 years.

2 Pain in face:
- Trigeminal neuralgia – mean age of onset around 50 years, rarely starts in old age.
- Dental problems.
- Sinusitis.
- Giant-cell arteritis (pain on chewing).
- Post-herpetic neuralgia (look for post-inflammatory pigmentary change in a trigeminal dermatome).

3 Hemiparesis:
- Vascular disease.
- Space-occupying lesion.
- Unilateral PD.

4 Paraparesis:
- Cord compression – either vascular or space-occupying lesion.
- CSF infection.
- Guillain–Barré syndrome.
- Pressure from disc, bone or collection of pus.

5 Unsteadiness:
- Neuropathy
- Proximal myopathy.
- Cerebellar disease.
- Drug-induced.
- Cerebrovascular disease.
- Middle-ear disease.
- Myxoedema.

6 Rigidity/immobility:
- PD.
- Drugs – especially phenothiazines.
- Disuse.
- Joint/bone problems.
- Spasticity of multi-infarct dementia.

7 Asymmetrical weakness:
- Nerve entrapment.
- Motor-neuron disease (MND).
- Diabetes – mononeuritis.

8 Clouding of consciousness:
- Meningitis or encephalitis and sepsis at any site.
  - Raised intracranial pressure.
  - Drugs (sedatives, hypnotics).
  - Biochemical disturbances.

9 Coma:
- Stroke (large lesions in the cerebral hemispheres, small lesions in the brainstem).
- Space-occupying lesion.
- Fits.
- Drugs (sedatives, hypnotics, alcohol).
- Poisoning (accidental – remember carbon monoxide – self-harm, iatrogenic, rarely, deliberate).
- Biochemical disturbance (hypoglycaemia is the one not to miss – check the glucose).

10 Involuntary movement:
- PD.
- drugs (anti-Parkinsonian treatment, neuroleptics).
- benign essential tremor.
- vascular disease (choreiform movements and hemiballismus are usually due to stroke in old age).
- epilepsy.
- cerebellar disease.

Aetiological classification

Vascular disease

See Chapter 7 for stroke and multi-infarct disease.

Trauma

Fractured skull

Fractures are important if depressed as pieces of bone may damage underlying cortex. Diplopia may indicate a fractured orbit. Fractures through a sinus or the ear may allow entry of organisms and lead to meningitis; so prophylactic antibiotics are given. Fracture through the temporal bone can result in an extradural haemorrhage. However, a routine X-ray of the skull after an uncomplicated fall is not justified. If an X-ray is done, fractures are hard to spot, but always look for a horizontal line indicating an air/fluid (blood) level.

Subdural haematoma

This is commoner in old age because of increased frequency of falls and it is said that cerebral atrophy allows continued oozing of blood in to the subdural space. A subdural may be asymptomatic, cause mild unilateral weakness, intellectual impairment, fits or loss of consciousness. A fluctuating course or disproportionate drowsiness in a patient with a hemiparesis may alert the clinician to this diagnosis. Increased use of anticoagulants in old age [e.g. atrial fibrillation (AF)] exposes many patients to the risk of subdural bleeding, especially if prone to fall or drink to excess, or INR control is poor due to frequent changes in drug regime or poor compliance.

Diagnosis confirmed by head CT. The hardest decision is often whether to operate, and although the appearance of the blood alters with time, it can be hard to be precise about when the subdural developed. It is difficult to predict whether drainage will improve the clinical state, particularly in dementia. Find out as much in detail as possible about the patient's prior functional performance as possible from carers or relatives and discuss with a neurosurgeon.

Cord compression

Cord compression may be secondary to a prolapsed disc, pressure from tumour, osteophytes (especially cervical spondylosis) or collapsed vertebra (usually secondary to other pathology, from osteoporosis to malignant disease), discitis (which is vertebral osteomyelitis) or an epidural abscess. A fall may be the precipitating event in a patient who had asymptomatic pathology. Plain X-rays are sometimes difficult to interpret, especially in the cervical spine, where degenerative changes are very common.

A sensory level, if present, will help identify the region for further investigation; it is usually several segments below the level of cord compression. Remember that lesions in the lumbar region or lower will present with lower-motor-neuron (LMN) signs as the cord ends at L1/2 and those above with upper-motor-neuron (UMN) signs or a mixed picture, e.g. cervical spondylosis causing compression leads to LMN symptoms and signs in the arms but UMN changes in legs. Check for loss of sphincter control.

Sudden onset of cord compression is an emergency and rapid investigation is essential if active intervention (surgery or radiotherapy) is to avoid permanent damage. MRI is better than CT, but the latter may be preferable if it is available faster.

Lumbar canal stenosis

This is usually due to a congenitally narrow canal but presents in middle or old age as osteophytes or a disc encroach on the cauda equina; remember the cord terminates at L2 in adults. It may produce weakness of the legs or be present with a pain, like intermittent claudication (better on stairs as the spine is flexed).

Normal pressure hydrocephalus

Normal pressure hydrocephalus is a condition exclusive to later life. Its cause is unknown, but simplistically it is assumed that when the condition is developing some abnormality in CSF flow must at least sporadically increase the pressure. Its presentation is insidious, with a triad of intellectual failure, unsteadiness (with broad-based gait or gait apraxia) and early urinary incontinence. Diagnosis is made by CT, which will show enlarged ventricles without widened sulci. However, variation in the relative amounts of ventricular enlargement to cerebral atrophy in normal ageing and dementia make this a difficult diagnosis. By the time of diagnosis, the CSF pressure is 'normal'. Treatment by shunting may be successful and in specialist centres, CSF flow studies may be undertaken to try to improve prediction of outcome. However, the procedure is rare and as there are no trials, Cochrane concluded that there was no evidence to support shunting. Where there is benefit, subjects with short duration gait problems do best.

Hydrocephalus may also be secondary to previous cerebral damage from episodes of bleeding (especially SAH) or meningitis. A strategically placed space-occupying lesion in the mid-brain may also lead to hydrocephalus.

Degenerative or idiopathic disease

Parkinson's disease

This is an idiopathic degenerative condition with progressive death of the dopaminergic neurons of the substantia nigra (SN) in the basal ganglia. Symptoms appear when around 80% of the dopamine has been lost and are due to a lack of dopamine and a relative excess of acetylcholine. PD is thought to occur in the genetically susceptible exposed to an environmental trigger but the nature of both components remains unknown (chronic low-dose pesticide exposure remains an environmental favourite). Rare young-onset PD has a clearer genetic component and some of the gene defects are characterized. At histological examination (post-mortem), the finding of Lewy bodies (intracytoplasmic inclusion bodies containing alpha synuclein) restricted to the SN is pathognomonic. Many cases diagnosed in life, even by experts (perhaps 10%) are not confirmed as PD on post-mortem examination. The incidence increases with age (250 in 10^5 aged 60–69 to 2000 in 10^5 aged over 80). Patients can be encouraged to eventually leave their brain to the PD brain bank.

Diagnosis

Parkinson's disease is always a difficult diagnosis in the early stages, especially in the very old, who may 'normally' have some features of extrapyramidal rigidity. The triad of classical symptoms and signs are poverty of movement (akinesia, bradykinesia), regular tremor at rest (5/sec 'pill rolling') and rigidity of extrapyramidal type ('lead pipe') or cogwheel rigidity in presence of tremor.

The tremor may be obvious and is usually a rest tremor and may be unilateral. It disappears in sleep. The bradykinesia may be apparent as paucity of facial expression (Parkinsonian facies), and there is difficulty with fine movements, typically doing up buttons. The handwriting may get smaller during the course of a sentence (micrographia). Speech is soft (dysphonic), monotonous and becomes dysarthric. The stiffness may be misinterpreted as arthritis, and although PD does not affect the sensory system, the joint stiffness, particularly in bed at night may be painful. The gait is characteristic with a flexed posture, tendency to shuffle, loss of arm swing and impaired postural reflexes, which make the patient likely to fall. Stopping, starting and turning are the aspects of walking that pose most difficulty, and if a walking frame is needed, a

wheeled type is usually recommended. As the disease progresses, constipation, bladder instability and drooling may be troublesome.

Documented response to therapy may be helpful in confirming the diagnosis, e.g. measuring the time to walk a set distance (10 m) or to carry out a tap test – the number of pronations and supinations the patient can achieve in a minute, tapping on a desk, or inspection of handwriting (micrographia should be seen to improve). Diagnosis is clinical but a ^{123}I-FP-CIT-SPECT scan, which uses a cocaine analogue to image dopamine transporter receptors on the presynaptic nigrostriatal terminals, can distinguish PD (where the cells die so the amount of receptor falls) from essential tremor (appearance resembles healthy controls).

Management

All patients with PD benefit from a multi-disciplinary package of care of which drug treatment is only one component. As the disease progresses the relative emphasis of the components will change. Learn the following list – suitably modified, it will provide an outline of how to manage most chronic conditions at any age, from multiple sclerosis to COPD!

Management options include:

1 *Education and support* – all patients or carers should be encouraged to join the Parkinson's Disease Society.

2 *Continuity of care* – chronic progressive diseases are best managed in settings that allow continuity of care to enable the patient and clinician to develop a working relationship and to assess the benefits and side-effects of treatment. In many areas there is a PD clinic run by a geriatrician, neurologist or both, often with a nurse specialist. The nurse can often visit the patient at home and provide telephone advice between appointments.

3 *Therapy* – assessment and treatment:
   • Physiotherapy: work on posture, gait, and falls prevention.
   • Occupational therapy: maintaining skills, home modification, etc.
   • Speech and language therapy: speech production, facial expression, swallowing.

4 *Dietitian* – advice on maintaining nutrition and protein spacing.

5 Assessment of benefits.

6 *Legal advice* – patients should be informed about lasting power of attorney and driving regulations, and may wish to consider living wills, etc.

7 Maintenance of general health and fitness.

8 *Treat other problems* – cataracts or in-growing toenails (refer for podiatry) do not help Parkinsonian gait.

9 Maintenance of *morale and mood* (consider complementary medicine, antidepressants; support from a clinical psychologist is rarely available).

Drugs

In the future, it is hoped to find 'neuroprotective' drugs that prevent cell death. Increasing evidence suggests that in PD neurons die by a process called apoptosis, which may be triggered by mitochondrial impairment and oxidative stress. Some of the current drugs, e.g. selegiline, may be neuroprotective but these claims are controversial. Several drugs now in trials have looked promising in animal studies. There is some evidence for benefit for co-enzyme Q10, a supplement available in health shops, but larger trials are needed.

Current drug treatment aims to restore transmitter balance in the basal ganglia. Whilst the classes of drugs available are logical (Figure 8.1), the order in which they are used varies not only with the patient but also the prescriber, i.e. the weight of evidence does not clearly support one course of action. Details of drugs used in the managment of PD are given in Table 8.1. Assuming the diagnosis is correct, levodopa preparations usually provide excellent benefits initially, but over a few years, the 'long-term levodopa syndrome' emerges. Problems may be predictable at first. For example, soon after a dose there may be involuntary movements (peak-dose dyskinesia), and as the next dose becomes due, the effect of the previous dose may wear off so that the patient becomes rigid, immobile and frozen or 'off'. These effects can be ameliorated by careful juggling of doses and timing, but eventually the fluctuations can become severe, apparently random and the patient may alternate between

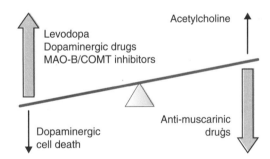

Strategies for dopamine deficiency
• Boost neurotransmission in remaining cells
• Reduce breakdown of endogenous neurotransmitter
 –MAO-B inhibitor
 –COMT inhibitor
• Act directly on post-synaptic receptor
• Most effect on bradykinesia and rigidity, turning the stiff immobile patient 'on'.

Strategies for relative acetylcholine excess
• Anti-muscarinic drugs
• Most effect on tremor, but benefit/side-effect ratio less favourable, especially in the old

Figure 8.1 Strategies for treating the transmitter imbalance in PD.

Table 8.1 Drug management of Parkinson's disease.

Mechanism	Name	Prescription tips (see BNF section 4.9)
Replenish striatal dopamine	Levodopa with peripheral dopa-decarboxylase inhibitor as Sinemet® (co-careldopa) or Madopar® (co-beneldopa)	Start low, increase slowly balancing response with side-effects, with meals initially to reduce nausea, later before meals as drug competes for absorption with amino acids from a protein meal. Can use slow-release preparation from the start or to cover the night, dispersible preparation if swallowing a problem. About 85% of patients respond to levodopa.
Catechol-O-methyltransferase inhibitor	Entacapone tolcapone	Entacapone, used with levodopa to reduce end of dose deterioration, may colour the urine red. Tolcapone only used if entacapone unsuitable as tolcapone occasionally causes severe hepatotoxicity.
Monoamine-oxidase-B	Selegiline, rasagiline	Used as early monotherapy or with levodopa to reduce end of dose deterioration. Concern (inconclusive) that selegiline increases mortality, led to sublingual preparation to avoid first-pass, reducing amphetamine-related metabolites. Give in the morning as a mild stimulant. Rasagiline, once a day, may be better as metabolites are not amphetamines.
Dopamine agonists	All need very gradual dose escalation as hypotension can occur in the first few days. The therapeutic effect is mediated via the D2 receptor; other effects depend partly on their activity at other dopaminergic receptors and whether they are derived from ergot. May be neuroprotective.	
	Ergoline family: • Bromocriptine • Lisuride • Pergolide • Cabergoline	Bromocriptine was the first but is little used in the elderly due to side-effects. Lisuride and pergolide can be used alone or with levodopa. Cabergoline is the longest acting, but is not licensed for monotherapy. All rarely cause retroperitoneal fibrosis and pergolide and cabergoline may cause heart valve problems.
	Non-ergoline: • Ropinerole • Pramipexole • Rotigotine • Apomorphine	Ropinerole and pramipexole licensed for monotherapy or with levodopa. Eye checks recommended with pramipexole so ropinerole gaining market share. Rotigotine, delivered via a patch for monotherapy in early PD. Apomorphine can only be used subcutaneously; given via a pen or pump under specialist supervision for intractable fluctuations.
Antimuscarinic drugs	Orphenadrine Benzatropine Procyclidine Trihexphenidyl	Little to choose between drugs. Rarely used in elderly as worsen cognition, GI side-effects and urine retention. Used for drug-induced PD, tremor and may help drooling.

Notes: If nausea is a problem, give domperidone. Combinations may help compliance, e.g. levodopa and carbidopa plus entacapone. If a neuroleptic is needed, clozapine appears best but has restricted prescription; quetiapine is the current recommendation. Whenever any other dopaminergic agent is added to levodopa, reduce the dose of levodopa. If a PD patient is nil by mouth for any reason other than 'gut failure' put down a nasogastric tube to keep giving the drugs. All dopaminergic drugs should be withdrawn gradually to avoid neuroleptic malignant syndrome (life-threatening fever, unstable BP and rigidity). All dopaminergic drugs and advanced PD itself can cause sudden sleepiness, so warn drivers.

being 'on' for short periods only, with 'offs' and disabling dyskinesias. There is some evidence that the duration or dose × years of levodopa treatment affects the development of this syndrome, perhaps because of pulsatile stimulation of the receptors. In younger patients, long-acting agonists were increasingly used as the first-line drugs, but emerging side-effects with the ergot-derived agonists have reduced the range of drugs commonly prescribed. In frail older people, if PD is already impacting on function when the diagnosis is made, many doctors start with levodopa. In this group, the dose of levodopa is often limited by neuropsychiatric problems (confusion, ˙ hallucinations). Younger patients tolerate bigger doses without confusion, but dyskinesias tend to become more troublesome with time. The development of a transdermal drug delivery system is an attractive option for treating PD. However, local skin reactions are common with the first drug to be available this way, a rotigotine patch. Two other drug approaches under investigation are adenosine A (2A) receptor antagonists (e.g. istradefylline) and glutamate a-amino-3-hydroxy-5-methylisox azole-4-propionic acid receptor (AMPA) receptor antagonists (e.g. talampanel).

Associated problems relating to bladder, bowels, digestion, sleep and mood often complicate PD. It is debatable as to whether these are due to PD or common accompaniments to chronic disease and disability. It does not matter to the patients, but all such problems need to be helped by lifestyle changes or drug treatment. Although in theory SSRIs could worsen PD, they are used (but with extra caution if the patient is a MAO-B inhibitor).

The most significant complication of PD is the associated dementia, which is common in elderly patients. Rivastigmine may be helpful. Confusion may limit the patient's ability to continue with levodopa treatment. Neurologists once told Parkinson's patients that they would die with PD, not from it. However, the terminal stages of PD in old age are distressing, the patient being robbed of mobility, cognitive function, swallowing and sphincter control. Enormous amounts of support to both carers and patients are required at this distressing stage.

Invasive treatment in PD

More invasive forms of treatment are offered in a few specialist centres, but are not usually recommended for/available to frail older patients. These include neurosurgery – pallidotomy (for contralateral dyskinesias) has seen a resurgence. Deep-brain stimulation is gaining favour and may help severe tremor. Transplantation with fetal adrenal tissue did not fulfil expectations but may eventually become a reality with cultured cells, once fundamental issues such as how to 'turn off' dopamine production from transplanted cells have been solved. Trials infusing glial cell-line derived nerve growth factor (GDNF) were stopped amid controversy as to whether brain damage resulted. The first stage 1 trials of gene therapy took place in 2006. In two studies, the desired genes (glutamic acid decarboxylase, which makes GABA and neurturin, a growth factor that is closely related to GDNF), were inserted into the common adeno-associated virus that readily infects humans but does not cause disease.

Parkinsonism

There are a number of causes for a Parkinsonian syndrome:

1 *Drugs* – the most frequent being the neuroleptics, the saddest of which is prochloperazine; Parkinsonism is a devastating sequel to a usually ineffectual prescription for 'dizziness'. Some patients with drug-induced Parkinsonism have subclinical nigral pathology which becomes clinically evident when dopamine blockers are prescribed. Imaging of dopamine transporter receptors with SPECT can help to identify such patient; if the SPECT scan is abnormal the patient will respond to levodopa therapy.

2 *Virus* – post-encephalitic.

3 *Toxins* – PD induced by contaminated illegal drugs – MPTP (1-methyl-4-phenyl-1,2,3,4-tetrahydropyridine) and, more worryingly, case reports associated with Ecstasy.

4 *Trauma* – as in ex-boxers.

5 *Vascular disease* – the final stage of multi-infarct dementia, i.e. rigidity with dementia (this has

gradually been accepted by most neurologists as a cause of Parkinsonism). The gait is shuffling (*marche à petits pas*) but without the forward shift of the center of gravity seen in PD, sometimes referred to as 'lower body Parkinsonism'.

Parkinsonism often responds badly to standard PD treatments and the patient's condition may sometimes be worsened by such interventions, increased confusion and falls secondary to postural hypotension being the most likely problems.

Conditions allied to PD

Benign essential tremor

Formerly known as senile tremor, it can be mistaken for the pill-rolling tremor of PD but other Parkinsonian features are absent. Some cases are familial. It is usually present at rest and worsened by stress. It may respond to small doses of alcohol or beta-blockers.

Restless legs syndrome (Ekbom's syndrome)

This is characterized by a profound desire to move the legs and motor restlessness, which is worse at night. The dopamine agonists ropinirole and pramipexole taken before bed are now licensed for severe cases.

Progressive supranuclear palsy or Steele–Richardson–Olszewki syndrome

Extrapyramidal rigidity is of rapid onset, with paralysis of eye movement (initially upward gaze but not specific until other eye movements are involved). There is marked instability and frequent falls, pseudobulbar swallowing and speech difficulties and dementia.

Dementia with Lewy bodies

This is a syndrome in that Parkinsonism overlaps with features of AD and psychiatric phenomena (see Chapter 4). Brain pathology shows Lewy bodies identical to those in PD but scattered throughout the cortex.

Multiple-system atrophy, formerly Shy–Drager syndrome

Rigidity, with marked postural hypotension and other features of autonomic nervous system failure. Apart from attempts to maintain postural BP (avoid diuretics, hypotensives, keep hydrated, try TEDS , head-up tilt in bed, caffeine, fludrocortisone and midodrine, an alpha-1-receptor agonist), there is little else in the way of intervention.

Corticobasal degeneration

This is characterized by progressive nerve cell loss and atrophy of multiple areas of the brain including the cerebral cortex and the basal ganglia, corticobasal degeneration (CBD) starts at around 60 years. Symptoms may be unilateral at first and include poor coordination, akinesia, rigidity and dystonia. Cognitive and visual–spatial impairments, apraxia, hesitant speech, myoclonus and dysphagia develop and the patient becomes bed bound.

Motor-neuron disease

Motor-neuron disease (MND) is a degenerative condition of unknown aetiology that may easily be overlooked in elderly patients, where the UMN lesions may be assumed to be due to vascular disease. Most cases are sporadic, but around 5% are familial. In about a fifth of those the gene defect is in the *superoxidase dismutase 1* gene. In MND, mentation usually remains normal, sensory changes are absent and sphincter control is retained. The finding of LMN signs (especially muscle fasciculation) in conjunction with UMN signs is the most frequent clue to the diagnosis. There is no specific diagnostic test but findings on EMG/NCS may be very suggestive.

Patients with predominantly distal signs affecting legs and mobility often do well and there is only slow progression of their disease. Patients with an otherwise good quality of life and the form of the disease known as amyotrophic lateral sclerosis (mixed UMN/LMN) can be referred to a specialist neurologist for consideration of riluzole (a glutamate release inhibitor). This decreases firing of the motor neurons and prolongs the time to ventilation but is of limited benefit at any age.

Those with a bulbar presentation fare much less well, especially with the onset of speech and swallowing problems, of which the patient is only too aware. Such patients should be considered for percutaneous endoscopic gastrostomy to maintain nutrition and perhaps reduce aspiration pneumonia. The patient will normally be able to be fully involved in deciding on such a course of management. Do establish the diagnosis as many areas have a specialist nurse who can greatly improve symptom control. The MND Website has excellent information sheets for professionals, e.g. tackling excess saliva (sialorrhoea) and for the patient covering difficult areas like 'how will I die?'

Epilepsy in old age

After middle age, the incidence of epilepsy rises and exceeds that in children (children and adolescents up to 100 in 10^5 a year; aged 30–55 about 30 in 10^5; rising to 150 in 10^5 aged over 70 years).

Most fits in old age are secondary to cerebrovascular disease, i.e. up to 50%, only about 10% being due to space-occupying lesions. Other causes are sepsis, pyrexia, biochemical disturbance and drugs or alcohol (excess or withdrawal). Fits may occur in the later stages of degenerative disorders of the brain, e.g. AD.

Fits occurring in old age are usually partial seizures with a single focus of activity due to scar tissue following a stroke and may be simple partial (no impairment of consciousness), complex partial (in which consciousness is impaired) or a partial seizure, which proceeds to a generalized fit or generalized tonic clonic seizures.

Management

Investigate for an underlying cause. An EEG should be used to support a diagnosis of epilepsy; it cannot rule it out. MRI scanning is preferred to CT where available. It is usual to only treat after a second fit, but an antiepileptic drug (AED) may be advisable after a single unprovoked fit if there is underlying brain damage. Care is needed with AEDs; monotherapy is preferred, especially as elderly patients are more susceptible to adverse effects (including cognitive impairment and ataxia). Carbamazepine or sodium valproate are the first-line drugs. Check the rest of the patient's medication, both because some drugs increase the chances of a fit and antiepilepsy drugs have many interactions. Ciprofloxacin is not the best antibiotic in a post-fit chest infection because it is epileptogenic and care is needed with antidepressants. Rectal diazepam or buccal midazolam are recommended for urgent treatment of prolonged or recurrent fits in the community.

Fits may result in injury such as fractures because of underlying osteoporosis, and recovery may be prolonged by postictal symptoms and signs of weakness lasting for up to 24 h (Todd's paresis). The psychological and social consequences are at least as great as in younger patients. Patients and their families need a full explanation and education and are best managed with an epilepsy specialist nurse as part of a team, Think about safety at home – open fires should be guarded. Check whether advice on driving is relevant – do not assume that your patient is a non-driver.

Status epilepticus

Status epilepticus (SE) is a medical emergency with significant morbidity and mortality (>80 years mortality of at least 50%). The most widely accepted definition of SE is more than 30 min of either continuous seizure activity, or intermittent seizures without full recovery of consciousness between seizures. SE has a twofold increased incidence in the elderly and co-morbidity may complicate therapy and worsen prognosis. Acute or remote stroke is the most common aetiology. Non-convulsive SE (NCSE) has a wide range of clinical presentations, ranging from confusion to obtundation. It occurs commonly in elderly patients who are critically ill and in the setting of coma. EEG is the only reliable method of diagnosing NCSE. The goal of treatment for SE is to stop the fit activity as soon as possible. Usual treatment is intravenous lorazepam, followed by phenytoin, but if treatment fails, refer to intensive care for consideration of a general anaesthetic agent.

Infective diseases of the CNS

Meningitis

Less than 10% of cases, but over 50% of deaths occur in the elderly. Problems arise because of delay in diagnosis; the symptoms are more vague in the elderly, and signs, especially neck stiffness, are difficult to interpret because of the frequency of cervical spondylosis. Examination of the CSF is essential, but only perform a lumbar puncture after CT scan (papilloedema is frequently absent in elderly patients with raised intracranial pressure and fundoscopy is often difficult because of eye pathology).

The pnemococcus and listeria are common in old age and other atypical organisms must always be considered, especially in the very frail, malnourished and immunosuppressed. In the white population in the UK, tuberculous meningitis is more common in the elderly than in the middle aged. Ceftriaxone plus amoxicillin (to cover listeria), with dexamethasone is appropriate empirical treatment for bacterial meningitis until culture or PCR results are available. Steroids should not be given in septic shock and should be stopped if the LP suggests viral meningitis when acyclovir should be started.

Encephalitis

Headache, fever and malaise are followed by focal signs, fits and coma. Herpes simplex and zoster (particularly when a cranial dermatome is involved in shingles) are the most common causes. Consider the possibility early, as acyclovir is most effective when used without delay. EEG is helpful if it shows focal abnormalities particularly in the temporal lobes.

Guillain–Barré syndrome

This often occurs 1–3 weeks after a viral infection (respiratory or gut, especially *Campylobacter jejuni*) and usually takes the form of a rapidly ascending polyneuropathy. The commonest pattern in Europe and North America is acute inflammatory demyelinating polyradiculoneuropathy (AIDP). In other areas, an axonal neuropathy is most common. Motor features (flaccid paralysis with reduced reflexes) dominate but there may be some sensory involvement. By the third week of the illness, 90% of patients are at their weakest. Investigations include lumbar puncture; (CSF is usually cellular with high protein) and nerve conduction studies. Treatment consists of support, intravenous immunoglobulin or, less commonly now, plasma exchange and ventilation if respiratory muscles are involved. The Miller Fisher variant is characterized by paralysis of the eye muscles, areflexia and ataxia; a characteristic antibody anti-GQ1b IgG is present. If the initial progressive phase lasts longer than 6 weeks, this is termed 'chronic', i.e. Chronic inflammatory demyelinatng polyradioculo neuropathy (CIDP).

Poliomyelitis

New cases are very rare in the UK because of the polio vaccination programme but you will see older people with the sequelae – usually a flaccid wasted weak leg with absent reflexes (pathology is damage to the anterior horn cells). If the damage occurred in the teens or younger the limb may be small and a caliper is often worn for foot drop. About half the survivors (now mainly from the epidemics in the 1940s and 1950s) will develop the post-polio syndrome (PPS), which begins 30–40 years after the acute illness and is slowly progressive. Common problems include fatigue, cold intolerance, joint deterioration with pain, new weakness, muscle pain and atrophy, dysphagia and dysphonia, sleep apnoea and respiratory failure. The aetiology is unclear, but premature exhaustion of the new sprouts that developed after acute poliomyelitis appears most likely. Treatment is primarily supportive, although non-fatiguing strengthening exercise may improve strength over the short term. Drugs have not been beneficial in controlled trials.

Herpes zoster

Herpes zoster (shingles) is a reactivation of the varicella virus, which has lain dormant in the dorsal root ganglia since an earlier attack of chicken pox.

It follows that patients do not catch shingles from other people with varicella or shingles, but a susceptible person can catch chicken pox from someone with active shingles. Patients with shingles are often isolated in hospital to protect care staff. Shingles is particularly likely to afflict the debilitated and the immunosuppressed and may involve a dermatome where there is spinal disease.

Clinical features
• Pain in the distribution of the dorsal root with paraesthesia and hyperaesthesia usually preceding the rash by a couple of days, although the illness may be painless.
• The characteristic rash, like that of varicella, follows the sequence: papules–vesicles–pustules–crusts, and then ceases to be infectious. The dermatome affected is thoracic in over 50% but is trigeminal in 10–15% and, less commonly, the geniculate ganglion (Ramsay–Hunt syndrome), where a Bell's palsy may be the first manifestation.
• Anteriorly, the rash does not cross the mid-line, but posteriorly it follows the posterior primary ramus a few centimetres across the spinous processes. Sometimes more than one adjacent dermatome is involved but it is very seldom bilateral
• Less common features and complications include muscle wasting in the relevant segment, an internal rash in the same segment (e.g. the bladder), a mixed varicella–zoster eruption, meningoencephalitis and eye involvement.

Management
Attention to hydration and general health, plus aciclovir 800 mg five times daily by mouth or, particularly in the immunocompromised, intravenously, in the weakly evidence-based hope of minimizing the likelihood of post-herpetic neuralgia. Prednisolone 40 mg may be given, again with weak evidence. The advantage of famciclovir is that it can be given once daily. The pain may be severe and appropriate analgesia should be given.

Ophthalmic zoster
This requires urgent ophthalmological referral in case of corneal ulceration and with a view to local atropine, idoxuridine and/or aciclovir.

Post-herpetic neuralgia
Continued burning neuropathic pain for months or years afflicts more than half of elderly patients following an attack of shingles. It is often severe, debilitating, and intractable. This neuropathic pain responds better to tricyclic antidepressants, gabapentin, pregabalin or sodium valproate, or topical capsaicin rather than to conventional analgesics.

Malignant disease

Intracranial neoplasms

Metastases are more common than cerebral primaries. In 50% of the cases, cerebral metastases are solitary. Primary lesions may be amenable to surgery or chemotherapy, depending on site and nature – advice will be needed from neurosurgeons and oncologists.

Cerebral metastases are most commonly from lung or breast. Palliative treatment with dexamethasone will often be beneficial in both untreatable primaries and secondaries. The window of symptom relief will be of value to both the patient and their families and help them to come to terms with the prognosis.

Non-metastatic disease of the CNS

This is important in older patients (see further information at end of chapter) and may take the form of:
1 Cerebellar syndrome.
2 Peripheral neuropathy.
3 Myasthenic syndrome.

Deficiency/toxicity states

The B group of vitamins has an important role in maintaining neurological integrity – deficiencies can have central effects, e.g. dementia, and peripheral effects, e.g. neuropathy. Neurological complications may arise before other systems are affected, e.g. subacute combined degeneration of the cord may precede a macrocytic anaemia. In B_{12} deficiency, the findings depend on whether the spinal cord degeneration (pyramidal tracts and dorsal columns 'combined') or neuropathy dominate.

Always consider deficiency states (including myxoedema) that can usually be easily confirmed and, more importantly, treated. Toxicity and deficiencies may occur together, as in alcoholic abuse. The alcohol can have a direct toxic effect on the nervous system (central and peripheral) and also lead to nutritional deficiencies because of the associated malnutrition and poor intake of nutrients, such as folate.

Diabetes can also be included in this section, as a cause of peripheral neuropathy, either symmetrical or in the form of mononeuritis multiplex.

Drugs should also be included as a cause for many neurological conditions, e.g.:
- PD – secondary to neuroleptics.
- Ataxia – secondary to anticonvulsant toxicity.
- Tardive dyskinesia – secondary to neuroleptics.
- Peripheral neuropathy – especially anti-neoplastic drugs, occasionally statins, nitrofurantoin, colchicine, amiodarone.
- Fits.

Previous surgery may also be important, e.g. thyroidectomy, gastrectomy or ileal resection, the latter two leading to potential B_{12} malabsorption.

Entrapment neuropathies

Carpal tunnel syndrome

This can be mistaken for a peripheral neuropathy, as patients may complain of paraesthesia or dropping things, but it is due to compression of the median nerve in the wrist. Look for reduced sensation over the lateral palm splitting the ring finger, wasting of the thenar eminence and weakness of abductor pollicis brevis. Steroid injections may give temporary relief, but if there are signs of nerve damage, refer for nerve conduction studies and then surgery.

Meralgia paraesthetica

This is not serious, but if you recognize it, the patient will be grateful for the reassurance! It is entrapment of the lateral cutaneous nerve of the thigh under inguinal ligament, commonly in the obese, resulting in numbness and tingling in the anterolateral thigh.

Further information

British Epilepsy Association website – Epilepsy Action: www.epilepsy.org.uk

Collins, N.S., Shapiro R.A. and Ramsay R.E. (2006) Elders with epilepsy. *Medical Clinics of North America*, **90**, 945–66.

de Beukelaar, J.W. and Sillevis Smitt PA. (2006) Managing Paraneoplastic Neurological Disorders. *The Oncologist*, **11**, 292–305. Free full text online: http://theoncologist.alphamedpress.org/cgi/content/full/11/3/292#T2

Esmonde T. and Cooke, S. (2002) *Shunting for Normal Pressure Hydrocephalus (NPH)* (Cochrane Review). The Cochrane Library, Issue 3. Update Software Ltd, Oxford.

Guillain Barré Society website: www.gbs.org.uk

Guillain Barré syndrome: good online review of management:http://www.emedicine.com/emerg/topic222.htm

Howard, R.S. (2005) Poliomyelitis and the postpolio syndrome. *British Medical Journal*, **330**, 1314–18. Free full text online: http://www.bmj.com/cgi/content/full/330/7503/1314

McGirt, M.J., Woodworth, G., Coon, A.L., Thomas, G., Williams, M.A. and Rigamonti, D. (2005) Diagnosis, treatment, and analysis of long-term outcomes in idiopathic normal-pressure hydrocephalus. *Neurosurgery*, **57**, 699–705.

Motor neurone disease society website: http://www.mndassociation.org/index.html

National Institute of Neurological Disorders and Stroke website – a fantastic website with patient-friendly (hence student-friendly) material on a whole variety of neurological diseases you didn't know existed as well as the standard topics: http://www.ninds.nih.gov/

NICE guidelines for epilepsy 2004: http://www.nice.org.uk/CG020

NICE guidelines (RCP) for PD 2006: http://www.nice.org.uk/guidance/CG35/guidance/pdf/English

Nutt, J.G. and Wooten, G.F. (2005) Diagnosis and initial management of Parkinson's disease. *New England Journal of Medicine*, **353**, 1021–7.

Opstelten, W. and Zaal, M.J.W. (2005) Managing ophthalmic herpes zoster in primary care *British*

Medical Journal, **331**, 147–51. Free full text online: http://www.bmj.com/cgi/content/full/331/7509/147

Parkinson's disease NINDS website with good research links: http://www.ninds.nih.gov/funding/research/parkinsonsweb/index.htm

Parkinson's Disease Society website gives excellent, up-to-date general information: www.parkinsons.org.uk

Rao, S.S., Hofmann, L.A. and Shakil A. (2006) Parkinson's disease: diagnosis and treatment. *American Family Physician,* **74**, 2046–54. Free full text online: http://www.aafp.org/afp/20061215/2046.html

Roth, B.L. (2007) Drugs and valvular heart disease. *New England Journal of Medicine*, **356**, 6–9 Editorial accompanying 2 original papers showing increased risk with pergolide and cabergoline.

Savitt, J.M., Dawson, V.L. and Dawson, T.M. (2006) Diagnosis and treatment of Parkinson disease: molecules to medicine. *The Journal of Clinical Investigation*, **116**, 1744–54. http://www.jci.org/cgi/reprint/116/7/1744

Chapter 9

Cardiovascular disorders

Age changes

1 Reduction in the number of cardiac myocytes secondary to apoptosis, and hypertrophy of the remainder.

2 Accumulation of intracellular lipofuscin and extracellular amyloid.

3 Increased intercellular collagen, with reduction in LV diastolic compliance.

4 Patchy fibrosis of conduction system and reduction in number of pacemaker cells in sinoatrial node.

5 Reduction in adrenergic receptors.

6 Variable decline in stroke volume, cardiac output, maximum heart rate and maximal oxygen consumption. Many of these changes can be reversed by regular exercise (for the average 70–75-year-old female in the UK, walking at 5 km/h represents maximal aerobic exercise).

7 Lateral displacement of apex beat is a common finding and the cardiothoracic ratio on chest X-ray (CXR) is greater than 50% in 70% of women aged over 70, partly owing to chest distortion, due, e.g. to kyphoscoliosis.

8 Calcification of aortic valve cusps and mitral ring.

9 Dilated, elongated aorta and stiff vessel walls due to fragmentation of elastin: afterload on ventricle rises.

Heart disease

Types seen in old age

- Ischaemic.
- Hypertensive.
- Valvular.
- Pulmonary.
- Cardiomyopathy.
- Thyrotoxic.
- Conducting-tissue disease.
- Congenital.

Manifestations

See Figure 9.1.

Ischaemic heart disease

This is the most common cause of death in the UK and the USA. Over 80% of all cardiac deaths in the UK occur in those aged over 65. The sex incidence is equal, unlike in younger age groups. The risk factors are the same as for cerebrovascular disease; see Table 7.2, pp. 65–66.

Presentation

- Angina.
- Acute coronary syndromes (ACS): unstable angina and myocardial infarction (MI).

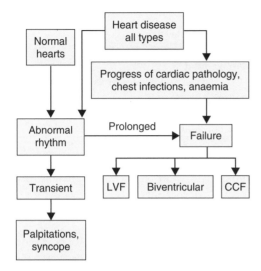

Figure 9.1 Manifestations of heart disease.

- Sudden death.
- Heart failure.
- Arrhythmias.

Chronic stable angina

Angina is pain secondary to ischaemia caused by reduced blood flow to the heart muscle secondary to atherosclerotic plaque. Stable angina suggests stable plaque disease.

- The classical picture is retrosternal pain radiating to the left arm and throat on exertion.
- The pain is reproducible by exertion, exercise and stress.
- It is relieved by rest or glyceryl trinitrate (GTN) spray, usually in less than 15 min.
- May present as breathlessness on exertion.
- If the chest pain becomes more frequent, lasts longer or is more severe, this is suggestive of plaque rupture, i.e. ACS.

Investigations

- ECG: may be normal at this point, or show signs of LV hypertrophy, or other evidence of ischaemia.
- CXR: likely to be normal, but may show cardiomegaly, or signs of LVF.

Management

- Address all risk factors (stop smoking, treat anaemia, hypertension and aortic valve disease).
- Aspirin, 75mg daily unless there are contraindications.
- Advise patient to take GTN prior to exercise.
- Commence anti-anginal treatment, for example:
- Nitrates (ensure nitrate-free period by giving isosorbide mononitrate modified release once daily or remind patient to take the patch off at night).
- Beta-blockers, e.g. atenolol, unless contra-indicated.
- Calcium antagonists, e.g. diltiazem.
- Nicorandil, a potassium channel opener, is a good choice for patients with low BP.
- A new class of drugs that inhibit the I(f) channel, such as ivabradine, look promising as they reduce heart rate without lowering blood pressure as beta-blockers inevitably do. Ivabradine is a selective and specific I(f) inhibitor that acts on one of the most important ionic currents for the regulation of the pacemaker activity of sinoatial node cells.
- In fit older people, consider benefits of cholesterol lowering agent, usually a statin.

Acute Coronary Syndrome

Definition

The ACS encompasses two groups: unstable angina and non-ST-elevation infarcts (NSTEMI), and ST-elevation infarcts (STEMI). This is because they are managed differently and they have different prognosis.

Unstable angina and NSTEMI

This is chest pain secondary to enlargement or rupture of atherosclerotic plaque. Features include:

1 Chest pain at rest or minimal exertion.
2 The pain is not relieved by GTN.
3 Crescendo angina on chronic background.
4 Angina of new onset on minimal exertion.

Investigations

- Serial troponin I measurements to exclude myocyte damage.
- The ECG may show signs of ischaemic heart disease: LVH, Q waves from previous MI, ST depression.
- The CXR may show cardiomegaly or signs of pulmonary oedema (see page 89).

Management

- Admit to a monitored bed if possible.
- Bed rest.
- Aspirin. Consider clopidogrel instead if patient is allergic to aspirin or has a strong history of gastrointestinal (GI) bleed.
- GTN spray/tablet.
- Intravenous GTN or buccal nitrate.
- Low-molecular-weight heparin (LMWH).
- Beta-blockers (atenolol or metoprolol), unless contraindicated.
- If not settling, add calcium antagonist (diltiazem).
- The use of intravenous glycoprotein IIa/IIIb blockers (e.g. tirofiban and abciximab, which prevent platelets from cross-linking and therefore prevent platelet aggregation) has not been established in older people. There seems to be increased risk of intracranial haemorrhage.
- Caution – watch for bradycardia and hypotension.
- Following successful management, reduce all possible risk factors and establish oral medication regime.

ST-elevation myocardial infarction

Increasing evidence shows that older people with acute MI respond just as well to thrombolysis as younger patients. However, several factors preclude this: atypical presentations (see box titled 'Presenting clinical features of MI'), late presentation to hospital, increased incidence of NSTEMI, which do not respond to thrombolysis, non-diagnostic ECGs because of left bundle branch block, etc., and the multiplicity of co-morbidities and contraindications. If the diagnostic criteria are met, the management should not be significantly different from that of younger patients.

Investigations

- As for unstable angina.

Management

- Give oxygen and opiates whilst diagnosis being confirmed.
- Stat. dose of 300 mg aspirin. Continue on daily basis if no contraindication.
- Admit to monitored bed.
- In the case of infarction with ST-elevation, thrombolyse with intravenous streptokinase. There is evidence that there is increased risk of intracerebral haemorrhage with tissue plasminogen activator (tPA) in older people.
- There is some evidence to suggest that older people do better with primary percutaneous transluminal coronary angioplasty (PTCA) because of the lower risk of cerebral haemorrhage compared with thrombolysis, but not many UK centres provide this service at present.
- Oxygen.
- LMWH.
- Treatment with oral beta-blockers, again to be continued if no contraindications, has been proven to be of benefit to older people.
- ACE inhibitors in patients with evidence of LV failure (to reduce LV re-modelling).
- Consider whether cholesterol-lowering treatment is indicated.

Presenting clinical features of MI

- 'Typical' chest pain (20%).
- Sudden death.
- Mild chest discomfort, sometimes attributed to indigestion.
- Abdominal pain.
- 'Silent', i.e. ECG changes or rise in troponin levels with no chest pain (up to 45% in the longitudinal Framingham Heart study), found in a patient admitted after a fall or 'off legs'.
- Heart failure, shortness of breath.
- Arrhythmias.
- Functional decline or confusion.
- A fall, found lying on floor unconscious, hypotension.
- Stroke.
- Peripheral gangrene.
- Post-operative fever, tachycardia, hypotension.

• Older people should have equal access to cardiac rehabilitation facilities post MI.

• If the patient is biologically fit, they should be considered for revascularization, either angioplasty or coronary bypass grafting. In this case, consider whether exercise or pharmacological stress testing is most appropriate. If no intervention is planned/ appropriate, then a 12-month course of clopidogrel is associated with a reduced risk of further events.

Heart failure

Heart failure is an extremely common cause of hospital admissions, readmissions, reduced function and institutionalization. Although often biventricular, it is conventionally divided into congestive cardiac failure and acute LV failure.

Acute LV failure

Clinical features
• Severe breathlessness, orthopnoea, paroxysmal nocturnal dyspnoea.
• Frothy pink sputum.
• On examination, there may be tachycardia, a third heart sound, crackles at the lung bases and, sometimes, pleural effusions.

Investigations
• ECG may show evidence of an acute infarction, LV hypertrophy, tachycardia, or left bundle branch block. Also look for AF, and other arrhythmias.
• Blood tests may show a troponin rise.
• In early failure, the CXR may show upper lobe blood diversion, fluid in the horizontal fissure or septal lines. With increasing pulmonary oedema, there may be perihilar shadowing and bilateral pleural effusions. If the effusion is unilateral, it is more likely to be on the right.

Management
• The patient is likely to be sat bolt upright already, but be sure to check as frail older patients tend to slide down modern hospital beds!
• Give oxygen via a face mask.
• Urinary catheter to monitor urine output.

• GTN infusion to offload right heart and reduce angina if present. Aim to keep systolic BP above 90 mmHg.
• Intravenous loop diuretics, i.e. furosemide.
• Opiates are very useful in this situation, as they not only reduce anxiety and pain therefore reducing oxygen demand, but they also reduce pre-load.
• Treat precipitant, e.g. fast AF.
• Exclude acute MI.
• Treat co-existing pneumonia with intravenous antibiotics.
• Consider short-term treatment with an intravenous inotrope, e.g. dobutamine, if the patient is normally very fit and independent.

Congestive cardiac failure

Prevalence
In people aged over 65, prevalence of congestive cardiac failure ranges from 5–10%, with annual mortality 10–50%, depending on severity. Frequent features include fatigue, functional decline, confusion, falls and cachexia.

Note: Ankle oedema is often non-cardiac – e.g. chair-bound immobility increases venous pressure, due to gravity, loss of muscle-pump activity and pressure on thigh veins by the chair.

Causes of biventricular heart failure
• Ischaemic heart disease is the most common cause.
• Hypertension.
• Valvular heart disease.
• Cor pulmonale including pulmonary emboli.
• Thyrotoxicosis.
• Severe anaemia.
• Arrhythmias, especially fast AF.
• Drugs, including non-steroidal anti-inflammatory drugs (NSAIDs).
• Cardiomyopthies.

Treatment
1 Advise the patient to reduce salt and fluid intake.
2 Stop smoking.
3 Control any abnormal rhythm.
4 Diuretics to reduce overload.

5 ACE inhibitor, unless contraindicated by poor renal function, hypotension or aortic valve disease (initiate in hospital in high-risk cases). If not tolerated, try a nitrate infusion.

6 Angiotensin II blockers can be used in patients who cannot tolerate ACE inhibitors.

7 Increase diuretics and ACE inhibitors as required/tolerated.

8 There is an increasing role for beta-blockers such as carvedilol and bisoprolol. They are now indicated for most grades of heart failure. They should be started at very low doses and titrated up as tolerated.

9 There is now evidence that spironolactone reduces morbidity and mortality in heart failure, and is often well tolerated in older people.

10 Treat causative or precipitating factors, e.g. valve surgery if indicated, hypertension, anaemia.

11 Digoxin for its positive inotropic effect in sinus-rhythm is probably useful in severe disease.

12 Anticoagulation is only indicated if there is a risk of thromboembolic disease.

13 Add metolazone to diuretic regime for massive oedema, but check urea and electrolytes daily.

14 Terminal stage – opiates and oxygen as required.

Diastolic dysfunction

Upward shift of pressure–volume relationship so that the normal LV volume and ventricular diastolic pressure is elevated. This pressure is transmitted back to the RA and pulmonary veins causing pulmonary congestion.

Think of it where there is a history of hypertension and the heart size is normal, and in patients with diabetes and infiltrative cardiomyopthies such as amyloidosis.

Current advice is that offloading with diuretics is detrimental; try low-salt diet. Avoid digoxin.

Hypertension

Definition

The definition of hypertension is constantly being updated. The current British Hypertension Society suggests aiming for an optimal systolic pressure of less that 120 and a diastolic of less than 80 mmHg. This is in line with the European guidelines.

Isolated systolic hypertension implies only systolic pressure elevated.

Prevalence

Among people aged 65–74, ranges from 45% to 64% according to different surveys.

Effects of hypertension

Major risk factor for atherosclerosis and thus stroke, coronary artery disease and peripheral vascular disease.

Effects of treatment

Up to age 80, treatment produces considerable benefit (more than in younger subjects) in total mortality and cardiovascular morbidity and mortality – but sometimes at the expense of making the patient feel worse. After age 80 there is as yet insufficient evidence to support treating all patients.

Treatment

1 Try non-pharmacological therapies first: low-salt, low-calorie, low-alcohol, high-exercise regime.

2 Drugs can be matched to other co-morbidities:
- Thiazide or loop diuretics/ ACEi/ ARBs for patients with heart failure.
- Beta-blockers/ calcium antagonists for patients with angina.
- Alpha-blockers for men with BPH.

Atrial fibrillation

Prevalence is about 5–10% in people over age of 75. The incidence increases markedly in those with biventricular heart disease and valvular heart disease.

Most common causes of AFl Ischaemic heart disease
• CCF
• Valvular heart disease.
• Hypertension.
• Thyroid disease.
• PE.
• Pneumonia.

Indications for aspirin versus warfarin

Aspirin for patients with	Warfarin (INR 2–3) for patients with
• Frequent changes of medication • Dementia • Tendency to fall • Uncontrolled hypertension • Non-compliance with monitoring of INR • Consider clopidogrel for those intolerant of aspirin	• Previous stroke • Mitral valve disease • Enlarged left atrium • Poor LV function • Controlled hypertension

---

Consequences

1 Reduction in cardiac output causes fatigue, lethargy, reduced exercise tolerance and heart failure.

2 Slow AF (due to digoxin or to conducting-tissue disease) may be associated with pauses. If only at night, these are not usually significant, but if symptomatic, may require pacing.

3 Systemic emboli, mainly to brain (stroke risk is increased by five times) and lower limbs.

Treatment

1 Acute onset, under 48 h:
   • Admit and give LMWH.
   • May revert spontaneously, especially if due to pneumonia or MI.

If persisting beyond 48 h, consider cardioversion, using direct current (DC) shock or intravenous flecainide, or amiodarone acutely or after 1 month's anticoagulation (to be continued for a further 1 month afterwards, together with maintenance sotalol or amiodarone to prevent recurrence).

2 Consider sotalol or amiodarone to maintain sinus rhythm.

3 Otherwise, control heart rate – aim at 90 b.p.m. Digitalization orally is standard therapy but verapamil or a beta-blocker in addition will be faster and more effective; amiodarone orally or intravenously (but central line usually recommended) also effective and sometimes restores sinus rhythm.

4 Exclude correctable causes – thyrotoxicosis and (possibly) valvular disease.

5 For AF of comparatively recent origin (1 year) without serious heart disease on echocardiography, which would make recurrence almost inevitable, consider referral for possible elective cardioversion.

6 It is important to consider anticoagulation for those remaining in AF. The risk of stroke associated with AF in the context of rheumatic heart disease is increased 17-fold and 2–7-fold in non-rheumatic heart disease.

7 Paroxysmal AF: digoxin is potentially harmful; sotalol or amiodarone reduce frequency of attacks and ventricular rate during them. High stroke risk: consider whether warfarin is beneficial or harmful on an individual basis.

Valvular heart disease

Systolic murmurs are audible in 30–60% of elderly patients and when significant arise from the mitral valve in 50%, the aortic valve in 25% and both in 25% of cases.

Mitral regurgitation

This condition is thought to be associated with some cases of transient cerebral or retinal ischaemia.

The commonest causes of mitral regurgitation in elderly people

• Calcification of mitral ring.
• Dilatation of left ventricle and mitral ring.
• Mucoid (myxomatous) degeneration of cusps.
• Floppy mitral valve with prolapse of posterior cusp.
• Papillary-muscle dysfunction – usually ischaemic.
• Rupture of chordae tendineae (often partial).
• Infective endocarditis.
• Rheumatic heart disease.

Calcific aortic stenosis

The triad of symptoms is angina, breathlessness and syncope or presyncope. The murmur may be unimpressive. However, if echocardiography assesses that the gradient across the valve is over 60 mm, and the LV function is good, the patient should be considered for an aortic valve repair or replacement.

Infective endocarditis

• The mortality remains 15–30%, with about 200 deaths in England and Wales each year.
• The majority of cases are now patients aged 60 or over.
• Previously unrecognized calcific valve disease is the major risk factor in Western countries.
• Dental and genitourinary procedures should be covered with prophylactic antibiotics, although it is not clear which other invasive activities should be covered.
• Patients with prosthetic heart valves require scrupulous prophylaxis for even trivial procedures.

Clinical features
The diagnosis depends on clinical criteria; it must be excluded in patients presenting with the following:
• Chronic fever.
• Weight- loss.
• Malaise.
• Intermittent confusion.
• New or changing murmurs help clinch the diagnosis but absence of a murmur does not exclude it.
• Splinter haemorrhages at the nail base.
• 'Classic signs' such as Janeway lesions and Osler's nodes are rare.

Investigations
• Raised ESR and CRP.
• Mild-moderate normocytic normochromic anaemia.
• Three sets of blood should be taken at least an hour apart from different sites. *Streptococcus viridans* is the organism most commonly isolated.
• Urine dipstix may show haematuria and or proteinuria.
• Transthoracic echocardiography.

• Proceed to transoesophageal echocardiography (TOE) if transthoracic echocardiography is negative and the clinical suspicion is high.

Management
• Intravenous antibiotics as guided by the microbiology department for the first 2 weeks.
• Oral antibiotics for a further 2–4 weeks. The patient will have to remain on intravenous antibiotics longer if the organism is only sensitive to vancomycin or gentamicin. In this situation, consider longer-term I.V. access such as a PICC (peripherally inserted central catheter) line.
• If the valve is badly damaged, the organism is resistant or if the patient is in refractory heart failure, the valve may need replacement.
• Advise the patient about the need for antibiotic prophylaxis for procedures in the future.

Orthostatic (postural) hypotension

Any fall in BP on standing up is poorly tolerated in older people because cerebral autoregulation is often defective, especially in hypertensive subjects. The definition is a fall of 20 mm or more in systolic BP or 10mm diastolic BP (prevalence 20–30% of community-living elderly people). It may be an incidental finding, and is only clinically relevant if there is good correlation with symptoms or distress caused by standing up. Symptoms include dizziness, presyncope, syncope, falls and visual disturbances.

Investigations
• Repeated measurement of postural BP, especially first thing in the morning and after meals.
• Twenty-four hour BP monitoring.

Causes of postural hypotension

• Hypovolaemia due to salt and water depletion.
• Autonomic nervous system dysfunction (Chapter 12).
• Drugs – antihypertensives, including diuretics, phenothiazines, antidepressants, levodopa, vasodilators (including alcohol), narcotic analgesics, verapamil, disopyramide.
• Prolonged recumbency.
• Cardiac disease (e.g. infarction).
• Varicose veins.
• Addison's disease.

- Urea and electrolytes.
- Short Synacthen test (synthetic ACTH).

Treatment
- Correct cause if one is identified.
- Advise concerning sensible precautions ('have a bath with a friend').
- Compression stockings, preferably full-length. Abdominal bands less well tolerated.
- Medication – fludrocortisone (a mineralocorticoid), or midodrine, a peripheral alpha agonist.
- Head-up tilt to bed (20°) to reduce nocturnal natriuresis.

Syncope, presyncope, faints, funny turns

- Consider in patients with recurrent unexplained falls.
- There may be a history of recurrent blackouts, but some older patients with syncope have amnesia for the blackout.
- It is essential to ask witness about loss of consciousness, signs of tonic-clonic seizures and time to recovery.
- Cerebral blood flow is about 50 mL/100 g/min in older people but is lower in those with hypertension or atherosclerosis.
- Symptoms of cerebral ischaemia occur when the blood flow is reduced to 25–30 mL/100 g/min.
- Syncope can be difficult to differentiate from epilepsy. Cerebral anoxia causes myotonic jerks, especially if the patient is propped up by well-meaning bystanders instead of being allowed to lie flat to restore cerebral perfusion. However, an epileptic fit is usually followed by post-ictal drowsiness or confusion lasting more than 20 min. An EEG may demonstrate abnormal brain wave patterns suggestive of different types of epilepsy. See the section titled 'Epilepsy in older age', Chapter 8.
- Blackouts associated with vertigo, dysarthria and diplopia may be caused by posterior circulation TIAs. Carotid circulation TIAs rarely, if ever, cause loss of consciousness.

Causes of a single episode
Any acute episode which causes a dramatic drop in blood pressure, e.g.:
- MI.
- PE.
- GI bleed.

Causes of recurrent episodes
See Table 9.1.

Carotid sinus massage
- The patient is lying down with their head in a neutral position.
- The carotid sinus is massaged longitudinally for 5 s on each side separately, allowing 30 s in between.
- Contraindications: recent MI, ventricular tachycardia.
- If there is a suspicion of carotid disease, this should be excluded by carotid doppler before starting.

Indications for permanent pacemaker
1 Symptomatic bradycardia, pulse less than 40 b.p.m.
2 Complete heart block.
3 Asystolic pauses lasting 3 or more seconds.
4 Persistent failure, lethargy and poor exercise tolerance are indications for pacing in patients with atrioventricular (AV) block, especially if trifasicular or bifasicular.
5 AF with partial block and a slow ventricular response.
6 Tachy-brady syndrome.
7 'Chronotropic incompetence' (a failure to speed up to cope with exercise – elderly people are unable to compensate for this with a rise in the stroke volume).
8 Cardioinhibitory response to head-up tilt, or asystole demonstrated on carotid sinus massage secondary to carotid hypersensitivity.

Vascular disease

Abdominal aortic aneurysm

This affects 3% of people aged over 50 and causes 6000–10,000 deaths annually in England and Wales. If up to 4 cm, regular ultrasound screening is advised; over 5.0–5.5 cm, advise surgery (if patient suitable). If unoperated, it results in 5% rupture per annum if diameter is 5–6 cm, this rises exponentially if larger.

Peripheral vascular disease

Presentation
1 Intermittent claudication.
2 Critical ischaemia (rest pain, ulcers, necrotic or septic skin lesions), sometimes following trauma

Table 9.1 Causes of recurrent blackouts.

Cause	Subtypes	Result of investigation	Management
Carotid sinus hypersensitivity	NA	CSM causes asystolic pause	Pacemaker
Vasovagal syncope	Cardioinhibitory	Bradycardia on HUT	Pacemaker
	Vasodepressor	Hypotension on HUT	Advise patient to keep well hydrated, postural exercises
	Mixed	Both	Both of above
Situational syncope	Cough	Good history	Avoid situation where practical
	Micturition/defaecation	Good history	Avoid situation where practical
	Swallowing	Good history	Avoid situation where practical
Orthostatic/postural hypotension	See main text		
Cardiac ischaemia	NA	ECG evidence of ischaemia with symptoms	
Arrhythmias	Bradycardia/ pauses	24 h tape	Pacemaker
	Tachycardia		Antiarrhythmic
	Tachy-brady syndrome		'Pace and block'
Structural heart disease	Aortic stenosis	Echocardiogram	Valve replacement

Note: CSM, carotid sinus massage; HUT, head-up tilt.

or a haemodynamic crisis. Those of limited mobility may not give a history of previous claudication.

Diagnosis

Affected extremities may be discoloured, with trophic changes in skin and nails (hair loss sensitive but extremely non-specific), cool and pulseless, bruits over femoral, superficial femoral (frequent site of obstruction) or popliteal arteries. Elicit blanching on elevation and delayed hyperaemia and venous filling on dependency. Measure ankle systolic pressure with Doppler probe – should be 0.8 of the brachial pressure.

Management

See Figure 9.2.

Giant-cell arteritis

The features of this disease are given in the following box. The incidence is 10–50 per 100,000. Women are more frequently affected than men.

Features of giant-cell arteritis

- Late age of onset (mean age 70).
- Temporal artery biopsy shows – thickening of intima, giant-cell infiltration.
- Cross-over with polymyalgia rheumatica (Chapter 6).
- Headache, usually over the temples, sometimes worse at night.
- Scalp tenderness.
- Tender, thickened superficial temporal arteries.
- Constitutional – fever, weight loss.
- Occlusion of short posterior ciliary artery causing blindness.
- Jaw claudication.
- Pain in tongue.
- Functional decline.
- Anaemia, abnormal liver function tests.
- Very high ESR is strongly suggestive, and can be used to monitor response to steroids.
- If not treated, risk of extra-cranial complications.
- Stroke.
- Coronary artery involvement.
- Peripheral arterial involvement.

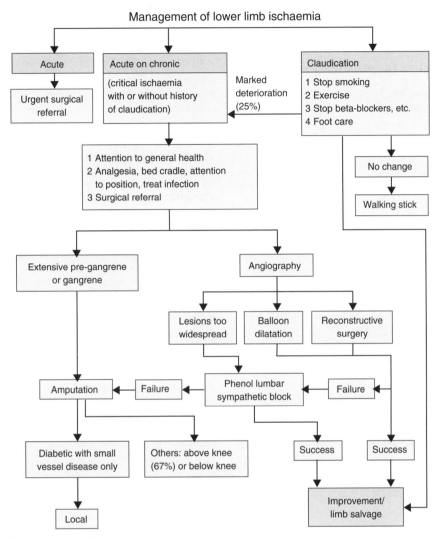

Figure 9.2 Management of lower limb ischaemia.

The response to high-dose corticosteroids (initially 40–80 mg daily) is dramatic. The dose is very gradually reduced to a level of 5–10 mg, depending on the ESR, and continued for 2 years. Remember to protect bones from accelerated osteoporosis, with a bisphosphonate.

Venous and pulmonary thrombo-embolic disease

Diagnosis of deep vein thrombosis (DVT) requires confirmation by ultrasound scan of thigh veins and,

if negative but strongly suspected, venography. Treatment of DVT in patients who are otherwise well can now be done as an out-patient with treatment doses of LMWH for at least 4 days, together with warfarin as per local protocol. PE is also treated with LMWH to prevent further thrombosis and allow endogenous fibrinolysis to occur. Once the diagnosis is confirmed, start warfarin. In the case of massive PE, especially where cardiac arrest is pending – consider thrombolysis.

Prevention is always preferable to cure: consider compression stockings and prophylactic doses of

LMWH in high-risk hospitalized patients, such as those with pneumonia or heart failure.

Risk factors for pulmonary embolism

- Increasing age.
- Immobility.
- Surgery especially abdominal.
- Fractures especially lower limb.
- Malignant disease.
- Obesity.
- Procoagulant states.

Diagnosis of pulmonary embolism

- ECG most commonly shows sinus tachycardia. Rarely there may be signs of right heart strain, or new AF.
- The CXR is often normal but may show segmental collapse, a raised hemidiaphragm or a pleural effusion.
- Blood gases may be normal early on but hypoxaemia is suggestive of PE.
- A negative d-dimer in a patient with low clinical probability reliably excludes DVT/PE.
- The mainstay of diagnosis is by isotope V/Q scan, except where the CXR is abnormal.
- If there is co-existent cardiorespiratory disease CT pulmonary angiography is extremely useful in detecting PEs. It has the additional advantage of demonstrating the true diagnosis.

Pulmonary embolism presentation

- Typical – pleuritic pain, haemoptysis (25%).
- Collapse.
- Sudden death.
- Fever.
- Breathless attacks.
- Arrhythmia.
- Cough, 'pneumonia'.
- Bronchospasm.
- Right heart failure.
- Pulmonary oedema.
- Increasing exertional dyspnoea.
- Confusion.
- Falls.
- Functional decline, hypotension.

Treatment of venous thromboembolism (VTE)

- Commence LMWH whilst confirming the diagnosis.
- Load with warfarin, aiming for an INR of 2–3. Remember, 'start low and go slow', and that antibiotics such as ciprofloxin inhibit warfarin metabolism and thus raise the INR significantly.
- Once INR within range, stop LMWH.

Duration of anticoagulation

- Calf vein (post-operatively) – 6 weeks.
- Idiopathic PE – 3 months.
- Older patients are at increased risk of haemorrhage with anticoagulation. Avoid concomitant use of aspirin. Those with history of GI bleeding are most at risk.
- The risk benefit of VTE versus bleeding must be assessed on an individual basis for those with recurrent PEs.

Further information

Beever, G,, Lip, G. and O'Brien E. *ABC of Hypertension*, 5th Edition, Blackwell BMJ Books, City Hospital, Birmingham, UK; Conway Institute of Biomolecular and Biomedical Research, University College Dublin, Ireland.

Bennet, N. (1994) Hypertension in the elderly. *Lancet*, **344**, 447–9.

British Thoracic Society Guidelines on Management of Pulmonary Embolism: www.brit-thoracic.org.uk/c2/uploads/PulmonaryEmbolismJUN03.pdf

Chalmers, J. (1999) 1999 World Health Organization – International Society of Hypertension Guidelines for the Management of Hypertension. *Journal of Hypertension*, **17**, 151–83.

Channer, K.S. (1996) Treatment of atrial fibrillation. *Prescribers' Journal*, **36**, 146–53.

Consumers Association (1996) The antiarrhythmic treatment of atrial fibrillation. *Drug and Therapeutics Bulletin*, **34**, 41–5.

Goodacre, S. and Irons, R. (2002) ABC of clinical electrocardiography: atrial arrhythmias. MBJ. 2002 Mar 9:324(7337):594–7.

Insua, J.T., Sacks, H.S., Lau, T.S. Lau, J., Reitman, D., Pagano, D. *et al.* (1994) Drug treatment of hypertension in the elderly: a meta-analysis. *Annals of Internal Medicine*, **121**, 355–62.

Lip, G.H.Y. and Blann, A.D. (2003) *ABC of Antithrombotic Therapy*. Blackwell BMJ Books, City Hospital, Birmingham, UK.

Mulrow, C.D., Cornell, J.A., Herrera, C.R., Kadri, A., Farnett, L. and Aguilar, C. (1994) Hypertension in the elderly. *Journal of the American Medical Association*, **272**, 1932–8.

Sever, P., Beevers, G., Bulpitt, C. Lever, A., Ramsay, L., Reid, J. *et al.* (1993) Management guidelines in essential hypertension. *British Medical Journal*, **306**, 983–7.

Staessen, J.A. (1996) How far should the blood pressure be lowered? *Lancet*, **348**, 696–7.

Swannell, A.J. (1997) Polymyalgia rheumatica and temporal arteritis: diagnosis and management. *British Medical Journal,* **314**, 1329–32.

van der Vliet, J.A. and Boll, A.P.M. (1997) Abdominal aortic aneurysm. *Lancet*, **349**, 863–5.

Chapter 10

Respiratory disease

Respiratory disease causes approximately 20% of all deaths if lung cancer is included and is the second most common reason (13%) for emergency hospital admission, after injury and poisoning. More people die from respiratory disease in the UK than from coronary heart disease. In Europe, five countries of the former USSR (Kyrgyzstan, Tajikistan, Kazakhstan, Moldova and Uzbekistan) together with Ireland and Malta are the only seven countries that had death rates from respiratory disease higher than the UK in 2001. Social inequality causes a higher proportion of respiratory deaths than for any other disease. Death rates for respiratory disease increase steeply with age, and 87% of respiratory disease deaths occur among people 65 years or older. The three main respiratory killers are respiratory cancers, pneumonia and COPD. Lung cancer now kills more women in the UK than breast cancer. Respiratory disease is a common reason to visit the GP – in 2004, nearly 1 in 5 males and 1 in 4 females consulted the GP for a respiratory complaint. COPD causes about 90% of respiratory disability.

Age changes

Physiology

Age-related changes affect virtually all aspects of the respiratory system. Structural and functional changes occur, decreasing efficiency of gas transfer.

However, because the lungs have huge reserve capacity, significant clinical issues only arise when an elderly person becomes sick unless, lung function has been progressively damaged by smoking or air pollution. Older people may have difficulty performing many lung function tests, but simple spirometry is usually possible.

1 Reduced lung elasticity and chest wall compliance lead to air trapping, a rise in residual volume and a fall in the forced vital capacity (FVC), forced expiratory volume in 1 s (FEV1) and peak expiratory flow.

2 Increase in airway size and loss of alveolar surface decrease the lung volume available for gas exchange and increase dead space, reducing efficiency of gas exchange. Premature closure of small airways results in ventilation–perfusion mismatching, contributing to an increase in the alveolar-arterial oxygen gradient. Arterial oxygen tension (PaO2) falls from 12.7 kPa at age 30 to 10 kPa at age 60.

3 Oxygen delivery to tissues (VO2 max) decreases due to age-related decreases in cardiac output and body muscle mass, as well as ventilation–perfusion mismatching and decreased alveolar volume.

4 Mucociliary protection of the lower airway is impaired.

Examination

Check the rate and pattern of respiration. Tachypnoea suggests a cardio-respiratory problem and this can be very useful if the patient cannot give much history. Cheyne–Stokes respiration, in which the breathing becomes progressively shallower, sometimes culminating in an apnoeic episode before becoming progressively deeper again in a cyclical pattern, is more common in the elderly. It is often seen in stroke but may occur in apparently normal individuals. Note the chest shape. Significant kyphosis is usually now due to osteoporosis (previously TB). The patient may forget significant surgery; thyroid and thoracotomy scars are easy to miss. The normal trachea may deviate slightly to the right around an unfolded aorta. Many older patients have basal crackles of no significance that clear on coughing. Conversely, if the patient has poor air entry, an area of consolidation may appear silent. A silent chest is a danger sign in airway obstruction.

After a fall, check for bruising of the chest wall and 'spring' the ribcage for fractures (pneumonia usually follows). Remember other systems associated with chest problems, e.g. aspiration in Parkinson's disease, and check for heart failure. Oxygen saturation measured by a fingertip probe is a useful bedside test. The admission CXR in an ill old patient is often difficult to interpret; usually taken AP or even supine (check for scapular lines), often with rotation (check relation of heads of clavicles to spinous processes), sometimes with the head in the chest and with poor inspiration. A subtle diagnosis may require a repeat film when the patient is improving.

Upper respiratory tract infection

Rhinoviruses (mostly picorna viruses) cause coryza, the common cold. This is a mild systemic upset with nasal symptoms, but older people, particularly smokers and those with pre-existing chronic illness, may develop lower-respiratory complications.

Influenza is usually debilitating in the elderly, particularly in the presence of chronic heart, chest or renal disease, or diabetes and may be complicated by pneumonia, especially due to *Staphylococcus aureus*. Everyone aged over 65 years should be offered immunization in October/November.

The influenza viruses are constantly altering their antigenic structure, so every year WHO recommends which strains should be included in the flu vaccine. The vaccine may cause a mild local reaction and hypersensitivity to egg products is a contraindication. Immunity takes 2–4 weeks to develop and lasts 6–8 months. There is evidence that immunization of staff is the best way to protect residents of institutions, and some hospitals offer free vaccination to their staff.

Acute breathlessness

The acutely dyspnoeic elderly patient is a very common medical emergency.

Airway obstruction

Most cases are due to COPD but a number of patients have long-standing asthma and late-onset asthma may be increasing. COPD includes chronic bronchitis, defined clinically as sputum production on most days for 3 months of two successive years, and emphysema, defined histologically as air space dilatation due to destruction of alveolar walls. There may be a reversible component to the obstruction especially in asthmatics who have smoked. The death rate for COPD has increased in recent years at a time when death rates for the three other leading causes of death, namely, heart, neoplasm and cerebrovascular diseases, are falling. About 15% of those dying from COPD have never smoked and air pollution is thought to be significant.

Common causes of acute respiratory distress

- Left ventricular (LV) failure.
- Pneumonia.
- Exacerbation of COPD.
- Exacerbation of asthma.
- Pulmonary embolism.
- Pneumothorax.
- Inhaled foreign body (stridor, choking).

> **Features of severe attack of airways obstruction requiring admission**
>
> - Not able to cope at home.
> - Already receiving long-term oxygen therapy (LTOT).
> - Patient cannot complete sentences.
> - Respiratory rate >25/min.
> - Pulse rate > 110 b.p.m. (unreliable in AF).
> - Peak flow <50% of patient's normal or predicted.
> - SaO2<90%.
> - PO2<7 kPa, PCO2>6.7 kPa on air.

Management of acute exacerbation of airway obstruction

1 Humidified oxygen: 24% or 28%, if CO2 retention and check arterial blood gases (ABGs). If a patient on oxygen becomes drowsy, remove the mask, shake awake and recheck ABGs.

2 β-agonist (2.5–5 mg salbutamol) by nebulizer using humidified air not oxygen as the carrier.

3 Prednisolone 20–40 mg daily (100 mg i.v. hydrocortisone if unable to take tablets). Elderly patients may have problems with short courses of steroids including steroid psychosis, CCF precipitated by fluid overload and unmasking of diabetes (as well as the well-known long-term complications).

4 Intravenous fluids.

5 Antibiotics (amoxicillin 500 mg t.d.s., clarithromycin 500 mg b.d. if penicillin allergic or if more severe, co-amoxiclav 625 mg t.d.s. initially intravenously if indicated. Treat as pneumonia (see below) if sputum purulent, patient ill or febrile, high WBC or CRP, or X-ray evidence of infection.

6 Antimuscarinic (ipratropium bromide 500 μg) by nebulizer.

7 Monitor temperature, pulse rate and respiration, oxygen saturation and peak flow.

8 Chest physiotherapy if secretions retained.

9 Consider DVT prophylaxis – enoxaparin 40 mg o.d. or TED stockings.

10 Aminophylline infusion if obstruction remains severe (not if on oral theophylline unless levels are available).

11 If the patient is beginning to tire and pH<7.35 consider:

- Nasal non-invasive positive-pressure ventilation (has replaced doxapram and a good option for patients who are poor candidates for intubation because extubation may be difficult).

- Intensive care for ventilation if above measures ineffective. Find out about the patient's functional status prior to this illness before contacting ITU to discuss admission.

Post-acute/chronic phase

1 Unless the patient is very disabled, stopping smoking is still worthwhile. Patients need advice, information and results are better with nicotine replacement therapy, bupropion or a new selective nicotine receptor partial agonist varenicline; refer to a 'stop-smoking clinic'.

2 A steroid trial (30 mg prednisolone for 2 weeks) looking for >10% improvement in peak flow is rarely done now; most accept this is a poor predictor of reversibility and use long-acting inhaled steroids.

3 Stabilize on maintenance regime of inhaled β-agonist ± muscarinic agonist (tiotropium is expensive but once daily and more effective than the older ipratropium) ± steroid, ensuring inhaler and spacer device understood by patient. Large-scale studies of combination inhaler therapy of salmeterol/fluticasone (1000 μg) b.d. or eformoterol/budesonide (800 μg) b.d. over 1 year reduce exacerbations of COPD by 25–30% in patients with moderate to severe COPD (FEV1<50% predicted) but these combinations are expensive. Prescribe salbutamol or equivalent as 'rescue medication'.

4 Consider supplying antibiotics and oral steroids for patient to initiate self-treatment of an exacerbation (with clear instructions).

5 Pulmonary rehabilitation programme for those with respiratory disability (exercise and nutrition).

6 Depression is common – consider an SSRI.

7 Domiciliary oxygen can be provided for symptomatic relief (cylinder) or if the patient meets criteria listed in the BNF (PO2 on air when stable <7.3 kPa) and will use oxygen for at least 15 h a day, LTOT via a concentrator improves life expectancy. The Home Oxygen Order Form (HOOF) can be completed by the hospital or GP.

8 Palliative care for end-stage chronic lung disease. In addition to oxygen, an opiate or benzodiazepine can relieve respiratory distress.

Pneumonia

The commonest organism is *Streptococcus pneumoniae*, followed by *Haemophilus influenzae*, *Mycoplasma* in epidemic years (every third year), viruses, *Branhamella*, *Legionella*, *Chlamydia pneumoniae* and *Staph. aureus* – especially during outbreaks of influenza. Prevalent pathogens and their sensitivities vary from one locality to another. It is often difficult to identify the organism, as elderly patients often swallow their sputum, but blood culture is sometimes positive. Presentation may be typical or atypical, with tachypnoea and functional decline. Pre-existing airway disease is almost certain to deteriorate.

Aspiration pneumonia is common in older patients with swallowing disorders or following an episode of unconsciousness.

Pneumococcal pneumonia has a mortality rate approaching 35% in elderly subjects. In addition to splenectomized patients where it is mandatory, frail patients with chronic heart, lung, renal, liver disease and diabetes should be offered pneumococcal vaccine, which usually provides immunity for 5–10 years.

Antibiotics are traditionally given intravenously in the first instance to those with life-threatening features, as well as those unable to swallow,

---

Features indicating life-threatening pneumonia

- Respiratory rate>30/min.
- Diastolic BP<60 mmHg.
- Arterial PO2<8 kPa.
- WBC>20,000×109/L or <4000×109/L.
- Multiple lobes affected on CXR.
- Confusion*.
- Blood urea>7 mmol/L*.
- Serum albumin<35 g/L*.
- Co-morbidity, e.g. diabetes, heart disease.

*Very common non-specific findings in sick old people – in whom all pneumonia is life threatening.

---

although there is little evidence of greater effectiveness by this route. The regime in adults has usually included a second-generation cephalosporin, such as cefotaxime, but many hospitals discourage cephalosporin use in older people, as they are strongly associated with the often serious (for the patient) and always disruptive (for the hospital ward) complication of *Clostridium difficile* colitis.

In older people, a recommended regime for severe community-acquired pneumonia is:
- Benzylpenicillin 1.2 g q.d.s. plus ciprofloxacin 200 mg b.d. i.v.,
- Add flucloxacillin 1 g q.d.s. after flu.
- Add metronidazole 500 mg i.v. t.d.s. if aspiration is suspected.

Remember to reduce the dose of ciprofloxacin in renal impairment, watch the INR if anticoagulated and swap to oral as soon as possible as it is very expensive intravenously and well absorbed orally. Less severe pneumonia may be treated with amoxicillin 500 mg t.d.s. and clarithromycin 500 mg b.d.

Other measures include oxygen (same precautions as in airway obstruction), intravenous fluids, physiotherapy for retained secretions, relief of bronchospasm if prominent and nutritional supplements if cachectic.

Pulmonary tuberculosis

Despite repeated warnings in the international literature, the authors have yet to see a resurgence in pulmonary tuberculosis (TB) in elderly patients within their geographically and perhaps socially limited practice – even among patients on long-term steroids. Look out for the signs and X-ray findings of TB from the pre-drug era (chest deformity from thoracoplasty, scars in neck from TB node removal, phrenic crush or artificial pneumothorax, the common findings of apical calcification, granuloma and calcified lymph nodes or more rarely 'balls' on the CXR (plombage). Haemoptysis may indicate recrudescence of TB or a complication, such as the development of a fungus ball (aspergilloma) in an old cavity. Remain alert to the possibility of TB (especially in elderly immigrants from the Indian subcontinent and in conurbations especially London). Infections with atypical mycobacteria occur in damaged lung and immunosuppressed patients.

Isolate patients with suspected TB and productive cough until the sputum smear microscopy has been found negative for acid-fast bacilli (AFB). Send three sputum samples for AFB and request a radiology and chest opinion if TB is possible. Bronchoscopy and lavage may be needed to obtain sputum. Start treatment without waiting for culture results if the patient has clinical signs and symptoms of TB and complete treatment even if culture results are negative. The standard regimen is '6-month, four-drug initial regimen' of 2 months of isoniazid, rifampicin, pyrazinamide and ethambutol, followed by 4 months of isoniazid and rifampicin. If your patient dies, send autopsy samples for culture if respiratory TB was a possibility.

Pleural effusion

Common causes of pleural effusion

- Heart failure.
- Pneumonia – empyema often presents atypically.
- Pulmonary embolism.
- Malignancy (1° or 2°) – especially if 'white-out' on CXR.

Effusions are classified as an exudate (protein>30 g/L) or transudate, but this can be less clear cut in an elderly patient with a low serum albumin. Unless there is obvious heart failure, when it is sensible to monitor the response to diuretics, diagnostic aspiration is usually necessary and therapeutic aspiration may be needed to relieve breathlessness from a huge effusion. Seek advice about pleurodesis in malignancy and irradiating the track to prevent seeding in mesothelioma.

Bronchiectasis

Bronchiectasis, abnormal irreversible dilatation of the muscular and elastic walls of the bronchi resulting in chronic infection, is usually post-infectious (measles, whooping cough or TB) in this age group. The features and treatment overlap with recurrent

chest infections and COPD; physiotherapy and postural drainage are particularly important. Azithromycin may be useful.

Chest trauma

- Rib fracture – common after mild trauma, e.g. coughing fit.
- *Diagnosis* – local tenderness and pain on springing chest.
- Complications – shallow breathing and reluctance to cough may cause sputum retention and segmental collapse. Pneumo- or haemothorax: refer for usual treatment.
- Treatment – adequate regular analgesia (e.g. paracetamol, an NSAID with gut protection and meptazinol or tramadol), usually with physiotherapy, is essential to avoid infection. If associated with minor trauma, treat long-term for osteoporosis.

Carcinoma of the bronchus

This is the commonest life-threatening cancer in the West. In Europe, the age-standardized incidence is falling in men but stable in females. It has become mainly a disease of older people (75% of cases aged over 60 in one series, 66% aged over 65 in another) and in the UK of social disadvantage. Lung cancers are classified into two main categories: small-cell lung cancers (SCLC), which account for approximately 20% of cases, and non-small-cell lung cancers (NSCLC), which account for the other 80%. NSCLC includes squamous-cell (35%), adenocarcinomas (27%) and large-cell (10%) carcinomas. Adenocarcinomas are not smoking-related. Presentation may be respiratory with cough, haemoptysis, dyspnoea or slowly resolving infection (repeat CXR 6 weeks after pneumonia to check resolution) but is often late, with symptoms relating to distant spread or non-metastatic metabolic complications. Patients are managed by a dedicated multi-disciplinary team. After CXR, a contrast CT scan including the liver and adrenals is usually done before bronchoscopy for central lesions or transcutaneous biopsy for peripheral lesions. PET CT scanning with ^{18}F deoxyglucose is very helpful in staging patients.

In early NSCLC, pneumonectomy/ lobectomy remains the most effective treatment offering the possibility of cure if the patient is fit enough and lung function is adequate ($FEV_1 > 1.5$ L). Although outcomes have improved, peri-operative mortality of pneumonectomy (especially right-sided) remains high (7–23%) and there is major morbidity in 40% patients. Radical radiotherapy produces a few long-term cures. Chemotherapy sometimes offers worthwhile life extension (a few months). Radio-therapy offers useful palliation for superior medi-astinal obstruction, chest pain, painful bony metastases and haemoptysis. Early involvement of palliative care services (e.g. Macmillan cancer nurse in the UK) is important.

Small-cell lung cancer has usually metastasized at presentation and is staged as limited or exten-sive disease. Unless the patient is too frail, multi-drug platinum-based chemotherapy is offered and continued for 4–6 cycles if there is response, with radiotherapy if the disease is limited.

Malignant mesothelioma

This arises in the pleura and presents with chest pain, dyspnoea and bloody pleural effusion, as a result of asbestos exposure. Check for a history of industrial exposure – the person who washes the overalls may also be at risk. The initial course may be indolent, high-resolution CT scan may be help-ful but diagnosis requires pleural biopsy. Because of the association with asbestos exposure and the long interval between exposure and presentation the effect of strict industrial regulation will not be apparent for years. Mesothelioma is increasing rap-idly in prevalence, with an expected peak in 2015. It is important to diagnose; although management is palliative, compensation may be available – seek specialist advice.

Pulmonary fibrosis

The interstitial lung diseases are a group of disor-ders characterized by the abnormal accumulation of cells and/or non-cellular material within the walls of the alveoli. This results in thickening and stiffness of the elastic tissues of the lung, so that

---

> **Causes of pulmonary fibrosis**
>
> - Idiopathic (cryptogenic fibrosing alveolitis, known as usual interstitial pneumonitis in the USA).
> - Exposure – occupational, recreational or drugs (amio-darone, nitrofurantoin, gold).
> - Secondary – connective tissue diseases, sarcoidosis.
> - Focal – previous TB, radiotherapy.

patients breathe in a rapid and shallow manner. The thickening of the alveolar walls decreases the efficiency of the transfer of oxygen. Many patients are short of breath on exertion and some have a troublesome dry cough. Fibrosis presents with breathlessness, widespread or bibasal fine crackles and sometimes clubbing. The course is generally progressive but the rate is very variable, and some elderly patients will have had documented pulmo-nary fibrosis for a number of years.

Carbon monoxide poisoning

Incidence

- Accounts for 40,000 emergency room atten-dances in the USA per year.
- Attributed to cause the death of 50 people per year in the UK.

Clinical features and sequelae

- Carbon monoxide (CO) reduces oxygen delivery to tissues by two effects: it has an affinity for hae-moglobin 220 times greater than that of oxygen, and it shifts the oxyhaemoglobin dissociation curve to the left.
- CO also binds to intracellular proteins, causes activation of neutrophils leading to lipid peroxida-tion and may cause apoptosis in brain.

> **Causes of carbon monoxide poisoning**
>
> - Smoke inhalation.
> - Faulty heating appliances.
> - Poor ventilation of such appliances.
> - Deliberate inhalation of car exhaust fumes; less com-mon in older people.

- Patients are hypoxic but not cyanosed. The skin and mucous membranes may appear 'cherry red'.
- Mild exposure [carboxyhaemoglobin (COHb) <30%]: headache, lethargy, nausea and vomiting.
- Moderate exposure COHb 50–60%: tachycardia, tachypnoea, syncope and fits.
- High exposure COHb>60%: cardiorespiratory failure and death.
- CNS tissue damage can progress leading to neuropsychiatric problems up to 80 days post exposure, including Parkinsonism, akinetic mutism, as well as acute confusion.

Management and prevention

- The key is to think about the possibility of CO poisoning and to take an arterial sample to check the level of carboxyhaemoglobin.
- Give 100% oxygen via a face mask.
- Do not be misled by pulse oximeter readings: the pulse oximeter cannot distinguish between COHb and HbO_2.
- Consider hyperbaric oxygen early on in severe cases.
- Treat fits with intravenous diazepam.
- Prevention is obviously important. CO alarms are readily available. In the UK, landlords are legally required to have all domestic gas appliances checked annually by an approved engineer.

Further information

American Lung Association website – large number of lung conditions described in detail for patients and clear for students! http://www.lungusa.org/diseases/

British Lung Foundation website: http://www.lunguk.org/

BTS report, The burden of lung disease second edition (2006) http://www.brit-thoracic.org.uk/c2/uploads/finalproof.pdf

BTS guidelines for management of suspected pulmonary embolus (2003) http://www.brit-thoracic.org.uk/c2/uploads/PulmonaryEmbolism JUN03.pdf

Intute – an excellent gateway to selected medical sites – search for your term e.g. COPD http://www.intute.ac.uk/healthandlifesciences/medicine/

McGill, Virtual stethoscope: If you are feeling a bit rusty about examining the respiratory system and interpreting what you hear try the McGill Virtual stethoscope!http://sprojects.mmip.mcgill.ca/MVS/MVSTETH.HTM

NICE guidelines COPD (2004) http://thorax.bmj.com/content/vol59/suppl_1/

NICE guidelines for lung cancer (2005) http://www.nice.org.uk/guidance/CG24/quickrefguide/pdf/English/download.dspx

NICE guidelines for TB (2006) http://www.nice.org.uk/guidance/CG33/quickrefguide/pdf/English

Walker, E. and Hay, A. (1999) Carbon monoxide poisoning. *British Medical Journal*, **319**, 1082–3.

Chapter 11

Gastrointestinal disease and nutrition

Introduction

Gastrointestinal (GI) symptoms are common throughout life – and the elderly are certainly not excluded. Structural changes, e.g. hiatus hernia, diverticular disease and gallstones, all increase with increasing age. Functional changes also increase, e.g. motility problems in the oesophagus and large bowel, and falling acid secretion in the stomach. Almost one-fifth of the patients presenting at a geriatric outpatient clinic will have GI problems.

Age changes

1 Impairment of sense of smell and taste.
2 Loss of teeth (see Chapter 15).
3 Impaired coordination of swallowing and oesophageal peristalsis.
4 Reduced gastric acid secretion.
5 Reduced pancreatic function due to duct and parenchymatous changes.
6 Increased development of diverticula.
7 Reduced surface area in small bowel.
8 Reduced large-bowel motility.

Weight loss

1 *Ageing changes.* There would appear to be a natural tendency to weight loss in old age (in contrast to the weight gain so common in middle age) due to a reduction in body-water content, bone loss (osteoporosis), thinning of connective tissue and the conversion of muscle to fat. However, those who maintain their lean body mass as they advance into old age have a better life expectancy than their shrinking peers.

2 *Systemic disease.* Weight loss is associated with all chronic disorders, e.g. chronic obstructive airway disease, cardiac failure, chronic renal failure and with malignancy in all sites. Undiagnosed poorly controlled diabetes mellitus, thyrotoxicosis and Addison's disease are other examples.

3 *Psychiatric disease.* The apathy of depression and the impaired insight and self-neglect in some demented patients will lead to attrition. The paranoia of a psychosis may make food unacceptable. The hyperactivity of some demented and hypomanic patients may result in weight loss. Alcohol abuse should also be considered.

4 *Iatrogenic disease.* Impaired appetite due to unpalatable treatment, e.g. spironolactone, or due to side-effects caused by toxicity or side-effects, e.g. digoxin and levodopa, both potentially causing vomiting. Antidepressants and erythromycin cause nausea, and ACE inhibitors cause loss of taste or an unpleasant taste. Diarrhoea due to misoprostol or antibiotic treatment.

5 *GI disease*:
 • Dysphagia.
 • Dyspepsia.
 • Malabsorption.

Dysphagia

1 Problems in mouth (see Chapter 15).
2 Neuromuscular causes.
3 Pressure on the oesophagus.
4 Narrowing due to change in the wall.
5 Epithelial causes.
6 Intraluminal obstruction.

Neuromuscular dysphagia

1 Ageing (presbyoesophagus). Uncoordinated oesophageal contractions or reduced activity.
2 Cerebrovascular disease including pseudobulbar palsy – see Chapter 7.
3 Bulbar palsy, e.g. motor-neuron disease.
4 Parkinson's disease. Akinesia complicates swallowing – may respond to levodopa and speech therapy techniques. About 25% of patients are affected. Autonomic nervous system dysfunction also common.
5 Myasthenia gravis. Rare but important, because of good response to specific treatment with anticholinesterases.
6 Achalasia. More a problem of younger and middle-aged patients but may be an aspect of presbyoesophagus.
Note: Nasogastric (NG) tube feeding is usually only justified on a short-term basis when recovery can be reasonably expected. Fine bore tubes should be used and only when the patient is aware of the problems and will, with help, be able to cooperate in this form of management – especially if long-term treatment is contemplated. See Chapter 7 for gastrostomy.

External pressure on the oesophagus

1 Pharyngeal pouches. All pouches become more common with increasing age. Zenker's diverticulum through the posterior pharyngeal wall at the upper level of the cricopharyngeus may result from inco-ordinated contractions. When large and full, it may hinder normal passage down the oesophagus. X-ray diagnosis is safest – endoscopy can be dangerous. Large and symptomatic pouches should be removed surgically and endoscopic techniques

permit operations on frailer patients. More rarely, pouches may also occur at lower levels in the oesophagus.
2 Superior mediastinal obstruction. Secondary to malignancy (usually carcinoma of the bronchus) may be complicated by dysphagia.
3 Dilatation of the left atrium, especially in severe heart disease, can lead to dysphagia. A simple CXR, in conjunction with clinical signs, will usually be sufficient to make the diagnosis.
4 Aortic-arch dilatation.

Changes in the oesophageal wall

Barrett's oesophagus and carcinoma

Death rates from these conditions have risen dramatically in the past 30 years:
• Carcinoma of the oesophagus: 3–6/100,000.
• Carcinoma at junction: 1.5–3/100,000.
• Barrett's adenocarcinoma: 0.3–2.3/100,000.
Troublesome acid reflux is a risk factor common to all three conditions.

Barrett's oesophagitis has a high rate of conversion to malignancy, up to 150 times the normal rate. Ten per cent of the cases have evidence of adenocarcinoma at the time of initial diagnosis. However, most patients die of other diseases. Regular surveillance is recommended in those patients who are otherwise fit: every 3 months for those with evidence of high-grade dysplasia, 6 months to 1 year for those with evidence of low-grade dysplasia and every 5 years for the remainder. Patients at particular risk of malignant change are those with a stricture, an ulcer or a segment greater than 80mm.

Carcinoma of the oesophagus is the most important diagnosis (incidence on the increase and twice as common in men as in women). Position can usually be well localized by the patient's symptoms, which are likely to arise when two-thirds of the lumen is closed. Problems with solids, therefore, are the first and most important clue. Barium swallow is safest for diagnosis and great care is needed during endoscopy because of risk of perforation (results of X-ray examination should always be available prior to endoscopy). Endoscopy allows biopsy when the nature of the lesion is in doubt.

Treatment

Results are generally poor but palliation is valuable.

1 Surgery – for lesions at the lower end.

2 Radiation – for lesions at the upper end.

3 Stent insertion – when other measures are unjustified; pain and complications with this method are common and obstruction is likely to occur at a later date.

Inflammatory lesions of the epithelium

1 Oesophagitis – with or without stricture, usually at the lower end and associated with hiatus hernia and acid reflux; therefore, long previous history may be given. Endoscopy is the best diagnostic approach and allows biopsy to be taken (essential if any suspicion of malignant change), and also enables recognition of Barrett's oesophagus (gastric mucosa in the oesophagus).

Peptic oesophagitis may be treated with antacids. H2 antagonists may be needed in resistant cases. Proton-pump inhibitors (omeprazole) now treatment of choice. Strictures should be dilated.

2 Oesophageal candidiasis – the frail elderly are at risk, especially those who have received antibiotics, use steroid inhalers or are immunosuppressed. The typical white patches of thrush are often (but not always) present in the mouth. Endoscopy or barium swallow needed for confirmation of the oesophageal involvement. Fluconazole is the treatment of choice.

Gastro-Oesophageal Reflux Disease (GORD)

• Passage of gastric contents into oesophagus.

• A common symptom is heart burn.

• May cause respiratory symptoms such as chronic cough or asthma and also non-cardiac chest pain.

• Proton pump inhibitors most likely successful treatment in conjunction with eradication of any demonstrated *Helicobacter pylori* presence, plus lifestyle changes (weight-loss and cessation of smoking).

• Only endoscope if treatment fails to relieve symptoms.

• Incorporates Barrett's oesophagus and adenocarcinoma and hiatus hernia.

Intraluminal obstruction

Impacted objects may include food (especially if not properly chewed), missing dentures and other foreign bodies. Cognitively impaired patients are particularly at risk.

Dyspepsia

1 Indigestion is common at all ages (30% of the population) and 2–3% of prescribed drugs are antacids.

2 In many elderly patients the symptoms are very vague and non-specific and diagnosis, therefore, becomes increasingly difficult.

3 The lesions potentially responsible for indigestion become more common in old age.

4 Late-onset dyspepsia should be taken seriously and investigated by endoscopy.

5 Helicobacter pylori infection rises with age (up to 60% of elderly people are infected) and should be treated if demonstrated by either biopsy, culture, breath test or antibody test.

6 Many of these conditions are asymptomatic, e.g. 20% of hiatus hernia and up to 50% of gallstones.

7 Many patients will have more than one possible cause for their non-specific indigestion – a therapeutic trial may be the only way of identifying the responsible lesion.

8 Endoscopy is the investigation of first choice (except in the presence of dysphagia) and very

---

Lesions potentially responsible for indigestion

• Hiatus hernia: 60% over 70 years of age.
• Peptic ulceration: 20% over 70 years of age.
• Gallstones: 38% over 70 years of age.
• Pancreatic disease.
• Mesenteric ischaemia.
• Carcinoma of large bowel.
• Carcinoma of stomach.
• Gastritis (especially drug-induced).

acceptable for most elderly patients – care will be needed with pre-medication in those with poor respiratory reserve. Endoscopic retrograde cholangiopancreatography is most helpful in elderly patients with biliary-tract disease, and stones, if not too large, can be removed directly.

9 Ultrasound examination is the best technique for suspected gallbladder and pancreatic disease.

10 Special attention will be required when treatment is started, for example:

(a) Metoclopramide – may precipitate or worsen extrapyramidal syndromes.

(b) Cimetidine can cause mental confusion.

(c) Aluminium salts should be avoided in constipated patients and magnesium in those with diarrhoea.

(d) Bile salts have proved disappointing for dissolving gallstones – side-effects, especially diarrhoea – can be very troublesome in the elderly.

(e) It has been suggested that long-term use of proton-pump inhibitors may lead to malignant change.

11 Many drugs cause dyspepsia; therefore drug history is a very important part of the investigation and assessment.

GI bleeding

Almost every recognized cause of GI bleeding becomes more common with increasing age:

1 Hiatus hernia with oesophagitis.

2 Gastritis – gastric erosions – elderly patients on NSAIDs have a sevenfold increased risk of bleeding compared with the same age group not taking such drugs.

3 Duodenal ulcer and gastric ulcer.

4 Carcinoma of the stomach (Fig. 11.1, p. 114).

5 Diverticular disease.

6 Ischaemic bowel disease, sometimes difficult to differentiate from chronic inflammatory disease, e.g. Crohn's disease.

7 Carcinoma of the large bowel.

8 Piles.

9 Colonic polyps – 40% incidence in people aged over 65 years in a post-mortem study.

10 Angiodysplasia of the colon.

Acute blood loss

This is particularly dangerous in the elderly as the resulting hypotension may trigger problems in other systems, e.g. stroke, MI and renal failure. Speedy treatment is therefore required: initially blood transfusion but with quick and ready access to surgical intervention if the bleeding persists.

Acute upper GI bleeding in the elderly often presents as melaena without haematemesis – endoscopy may therefore be helpful in locating the site of bleeding and mucosal injection may help to stop bleeding.

Acute and severe ischaemia may present as rectal bleeding – but the ischaemia may be secondary to other pathology, e.g. a silent MI – a full assessment is therefore needed.

Chronic blood loss

Chronic GI bleeding is the most common cause of iron-deficiency anaemia in old age (see Chapter 14). The bleeding site will be asymptomatic in many patients. Investigation is therefore problematic – examination of both the upper and lower tract will be required in most cases and the ready acceptance of a simple benign lesion should not prevent further exploration for more serious causes – if the patient is sufficiently fit and co-operative to undergo extensive examination and subsequent treatment of any pathology.

Suggested plan of investigation

1 Confirmation of iron-deficiency anaemia.

2 Confirmation of GI bleeding – faecal occult bloods now less commonly performed.

3 Endoscopy of upper tract – to reveal or exclude oesophagitis and gastritis, as well as definite ulceration and malignancy. Barium swallow/meal is more appropriate if dysphagia is a problem.

4 Sigmoidoscopy followed by barium enema to study large bowel – preferably as an in-patient in frail elderly patients to ensure adequate bowel preparation. CT of the abdomen is kinder and almost as effective in frail elderly patients or those unable to co-operate with a barium enema and

provide extra information about liver, pancreas and lymph nodes.

5 Colonoscopy if barium enema or CT is inconclusive – may confirm abnormality previously seen or reveal angiodysplasia.

6 Radioisotope-labelled red cells may be used to confirm presence and site of GI bleeding in difficult cases of brisk intermittent bleeding from unknown site.

Treatment

1 Specific treatment for underlying cause.

2 Oral iron supplements – ferrous sulphate if tolerated.

3 Transfuse only if haemoglobin is very low, e.g. less than 7 g, and patient unwell; take care if risk of congestive heart failure is present.

The acute abdomen

A difficult diagnostic problem at all ages, but even more so in old age. The mortality rate in elderly patients is much higher and may exceed 50% in some instances; there are four possible reasons for such depressing results:

1 Delay in presentation.

2 Atypical presentation ('silent').

3 Reluctance to operate on frail elderly patients.

4 Precipitation of other significant pathology during the acute episode, e.g. MI and stroke.

For pathology found in patients aged over 75 years undergoing emergency abdominal surgery, see Table 11.1.

Table 11.1 Acute abdomen – pathology in elderly patients undergoing surgery.

Diagnosis	Number	Mortality rate (%)
Strangulated hernia	115	16.5
Intestinal obstruction	103	37.9
Perforated peptic ulcer	22	40.9
Perforated large bowel	22	63.6
Ruptured aortic aneurysm	9	77.7
Biliary-tract disease[a]	22	
Mesenteric ischaemia[a]	10	

[a] Reduced numbers as some patients were treated conservatively.

Useful pointers in the elderly acute abdomen

1 Check hernial orifices.

2 X-ray for fluid levels, free air in peritoneal cavity, and distended bowel (e.g. sigmoid volvulus).

3 Check amylase level – about half the patients with acute pancreatitis are over 60 years of age.

4 Monitor presence of pulses and use ultrasound for detection of aortic aneurysm.

Note: Always consider the diagnosis of 'acute abdomen' in 'shocked', elderly patients, if supporting evidence is found on examination and emergency investigation; act quickly if surgical help is indicated.

Bowel ischaemia

1 Twenty per cent of the cardiac output is used to supply the GI tract – therefore, any significant change in cardiac output is likely to affect the perfusion of the bowel and precipitate ischaemia.

2 At least two major mesenteric arteries must be compromised for bowel ischaemia to occur.

3 Because of a poor anastomotic arrangement, the left side of the colon is the most vulnerable segment of the bowel.

4 Arterial occlusion responsible in 50% of cases.

5 Non-occlusive mechanisms (low flow) in 20–30% of the cases.

6 Venous occlusion 5–10% of the cases.

Associated factors/conditions

1 Embolization, e.g. atrial fibrillation.

2 Reduced cardiac output, e.g. hypotension and congestive cardiac failure.

3 Drugs, e.g. digitalis, oestrogens, antihypertensives, psychotropic agents.

4 Vasculitis, e.g. rheumatoid arthritis and polymyalgia rheumatica.

5 Hypercoagulability.

Clinical course

1 Mild:
  • Post-prandial abdominal pain, diarrhoea and weight loss.

• Mucosal swelling – 'thumb printing' on barium studies.
• Recovery plus or minus scarring (stricture).

2 Severe:
• Sudden severe pain – but may be 'silent'.
• Movement of fluid into lumen, vomiting, diarrhoea and shock.
• Ischaemic bowel wall allows bacteria to cross from lumen to peritoneum – peritonitis plus or minus septicaemia.
• Death almost certain.

Treatment

• Acute/mild – support and treat underlying cause to prevent recurrence.
• Acute/severe – consult surgeons regarding resection; supportive and symptomatic treatment.
• Chronic – small frequent meals; correct any nutritional deficiencies due to malabsorption.
• Peritonism makes laparatomy mandatory.

Diarrhoea

A very incapacitating condition in old age, especially if the patient is already disabled and immobile due to other pathologies.

1 *Spurious*, i.e. obstruction with overflow, must be excluded first by rectal examination, with or without sigmoidoscopy. The cause may be simple, e.g. faecal impaction, or serious, e.g. carcinoma of the rectum.

2 *Infective* – cultures must be taken and patient isolated while results are awaited:
• Viral – most common, usually self-limiting and supportive measures only required.
• Bacterial – antibiotics only justified if patient's condition is grave; in mild cases they may prolong symptoms. May be endemic in hospital (e.g. *Clostridium difficile*).

3 *Inflammatory* – Crohn's disease of large bowel most common chronic inflammatory bowel disease in old age; diagnosis by biopsy and barium studies. Radioisotope white-cell scan also useful for determining extent of disease.

4 *Metabolic* – uncommon but exclude thyrotoxicosis; some cases secondary to diabetic neuropathy.

5 *Iatrogenic* – antibiotic diarrhoea common, especially after use of cephalosporins; purgative misuse; gastrectomy/vagotomy.

Constipation

Fear of becoming constipated is an aspect of old age that is more common than the genuine symptom. Seventy per cent of elderly people have their bowels open once daily, 11% every other day and 14% twice daily. Difficulty in passing motions is of greater importance than frequency of defecation.

Causes of constipation are:
1 Faulty habits – low-residue diet, low fluid intake, lack of exercise and neglect of call to stool.
2 Poor appetite.
3 Immobility.
4 Drugs – analgesics, anticholinergics and diuretics.
5 Metabolic – myxoedema, hypercalcaemia.
6 Psychiatric – depression, dementia.
7 Functional – irritable bowel, purgative abuse (cathartic colon).
8 Pain – piles and fissures.

Management of constipation

1 Identify the nature and duration of constipation (small, hard stools are often related to low-fibre diet or dehydration; soft stools in a dilated rectum are suggestive of chronic laxative abuse).

2 Identify any precipitating causes, e.g. drugs, or bowel, endocrine or metabolic disease.

3 A rectal examination must be performed and recorded in the medical notes before prescribing laxatives.

4 If impaction is imminent – enemas are required.

5 If not impacted but a quick result is required – prescribe a stimulant (senna); occasionally an osmotic laxative (magnesium sulphate) will be required.

6 For short-term treatment (associated with acute illness) – ensure an adequate fluid intake and mobilize as soon as possible. Prescribe senna if stools bulky and soft; co-danthrusate/co-danthramer if stools small and hard in association with opiates, otherwise liquid paraffin and magnesium hydroxide emulsion (milpar) may be an acceptable alternative.

7 Review the continuing need for laxatives once the patient is over the acute illness. Only prescribe laxatives on discharge from hospital if need continues, e.g. prior usage or continuing precipitant.

8 For longer-term treatment – high-fibre diet, attention to fluid intake and exercise may be all that is required.

9 For longer-term treatment where non-drug treatment fails or is impractical – prescribe a stool softener (co-danthrusate) or a bulking agent (ispaghula husk).

10 For intractable constipation – try a combination of treatments.

11 For terminal patients on regular opiates – titrate co-danthrusate/co-danthramer against response.

12 The higher cost of lactulose can only be justified in those patients with chronic constipation in whom a bulking agent has failed.

Change in bowel habit

Alternating diarrhoea and constipation is always a worrying symptom. Carcinoma of the large bowel must be excluded, but diverticular disease or large-bowel ischaemia and irritable colon are more common.

Barium enema examination can be an ordeal in frail elderly patients. Best results are obtained if the patient is admitted for good bowel preparation and sigmoidoscopy before the procedure. Examination by CT is easier on the patient and performed as an out-patient procedure.

Faecal incontinence

1 Highest rates found in nursing homes at about 55% and 15% in residential care. Community rate in elderly people about 3%, of whom about half do not report their symptom to their doctor or nurse.

2 Spurious diarrhoea due to faecal impaction (sometimes beyond rectal examination) is the commonest cause, especially in demented patients.

3 Circumstantial, i.e. intestinal hurry plus physical immobility may lead to faecal incontinence. Treat underlying causes and reduce distance to toilet or commode.

4 Neurological or structural, e.g. paraplegia or rectal prolapse. Treat underlying cause where possible, e.g. surgery for rectal prolapse. If cure impossible – cause constipation with codeine phosphate and bulking preparations and relieve bowels at regular intervals with enemas.

5 Disinhibition and lack of insight, e.g. in dementia. Use bulking preparations and encourage regular toileting habits. In institutions facilitate recognition of toilet (e.g. large visible signs or brightly coloured lavatory door).

6 If all else fails, use pads and pants.

Absorption

1 Small-bowel function declines with age but nutritional deficiencies only occur when additional factors intervene, e.g. poor diet or ill health.

2 Causes of malabsorption in youth may also occur de novo in old age, e.g. adult coeliac disease.

3 Maldigestion is more common than malabsorption, e.g. due to pancreatic disease.

4 Bacterial change in the small-bowel lumen due to stasis or diverticular disease is common (10% of elderly people) and is frequently clinically significant.

5 Ischaemia is a special cause of malabsorption in old age.

6 Iatrogenic causes must always be considered, e.g. post-gastrectomy, alcohol and some drugs, e.g. biguanides.

Possible indicators of malabsorption

1 Weight loss in spite of good dietary intake.

2 Low serum albumin level.

3 Unexplained iron-deficiency anaemia (with negative faecal occult blood).

4 Macrocytic anaemia.

5 Osteomalacia.

6 Obvious steatorrhoea is uncommon.

Potential causes of malabsorption in old age

The investigation of malabsorption in old age is very difficult and unsatisfactory, but the following possibilities should always be considered and explored wherever possible:

1 Previous gastrectomy.

2 Small-bowel diverticular disease.

3 Altered luminal bacterial flora.

4 Pancreatic disease – causes maldigestion and steatorrhoea.

5 Adult coeliac disease.

6 Lymphoma.

7 Crohn's disease.

8 Mesenteric ischaemia.

9 Drugs, e.g. biguanides, cholestyramine.

Coeliac disease

This should no longer be considered as only a disease of childhood. Most cases present in the fifth decade and new cases have arisen as late as the ninth decade. In the UK, it now affects 1 in 200 of the population. In 25% of new cases, the patient is aged over 60 years. Not all cases have gastroenterological/malabsorption manifestations – see the following box.

Coeliac disease

Presenting symptoms in elderly patients:
Diarrhoea or constipation.
Apthous ulcers or sore mouth.
Dyspepsia/abdominal discomfort.
Fatigue.
Anaemia.
Bone pain.
Weakness.
Family history.
Neuro/psychiatric syndromes.

The development of antibody assays, endomysial and antigliadin, have made the detection of the condition much easier. The tests are done on blood samples and there is evidence of increasing frequency of positive results at least until the age of 60; beyond that age we have no further information. The endomysial antibody is the most specific, but the diagnosis should still be confirmed wherever possible by a small-bowel biopsy (biopsy negative cases do, however, exist as the pathology may be patchy). Antibody negative cases have also been reported.

The condition may be associated with other autoimmune conditions, i.e. thyroid, diabetes, primary biliary cirrhosis and Sjogren's syndrome. There is also evidence of association with neurological conditions including epilepsy, ataxia and dementia.

A period of treatment with a gluten-free diet should be tried. The patient will be best placed to decide if the inconvenience of the diet outweighs any benefit gained in feelings of general well-being. Any deficiencies found at the time of diagnosis should be immediately corrected. The prophylactic aspect of dietary treatment (protection from malignant change) is of less importance in elderly patients than in the young.

For main presenting symptoms in elderly patients see the box.

Diverticular disease

1 Very common and becoming more so.

2 Over 50% of elderly people have large bowel diverticula, rising to nearly 70% in the eighth decade.

3 Men and women are affected equally.

4 75% of people with diverticular disease are asymptomatic and require no treatment.

5 Of the 25% with symptoms, 75% develop diverticulitis (and 25% of these develop complications – which may include profuse haemorrhage).

6 Up to two-thirds of patients actually present with a complication.

7 Common low-grade symptoms are colic, bloating and flatulence all very similar to irritable bowel syndrome (IBS), but the latter is more likely to have extra colonic symptoms and apart from patients with both disorders (diverticular disease plus IBS) is more likely in younger subjects. About 25% of the patients have both conditions.

8 Low-fibre diet likely cause through precipitation of high intra-luminal pressures.

9 Serious complications requiring surgical intervention;

• Peritonitis.

• Uncontrolled sepsis.

• Fistula.

• Obstruction.

- Uncontrollable bleeding.
- Inability to exclude carcinoma.

10 Treatment options in uncomplicated cases – none are sure winners, but the following may be tried;
- Fibre.
- Antibiotics – rifaxim.
- Mesalazine.
- Calcium channel blockers.

11 NSAIDS are probably best avoided (may precipitate perforation).

Endoscopies in the elderly

- Techniques have been developing for almost 50 years with both diagnostic and therapeutic benefits.
- Age alone should not exclude elderly patients from this valuable form of investigation or treatment.
- 3% of endoscopy patients die within 30 days of the procedure.
- However, the risks are highest in frail elderly patients.
- National Confidential Enquiry into Patient Outcome and Death on therapeutic GI endoscopy noted (2004);
- 19% of PEGs (percutaneous endoscopic gastrostomies) were considered futile.
- 68% of ERCPs (endoscopic retrograde cholangiopancreatographies) were considered futile.
- 14% developed respiratory complications secondary to sedation or local anaesthetics.
- Informed consent was sometimes questionable i.e. in two-thirds of the patients with dementia or acute confusion.
- The procedures are not always performed by clinicians with documented competence.
- Clearly common sense, compassion and practical skills all need to be employed if patients are to benefit and not suffer.

Percutaneous Endoscopic Gastrostomy

- In patients over 50 years of age, 18% die within 1 month of procedure, 44% die within 6 months and 54% within 1 year and finally 73% within 2 years.
- Only 9% of PEG patients return to oral feeding, i.e. 90% have a PEG until death.

- Self-extubation occurs in 12% of patients.
- In demented patients, there is no evidence that;
  1 Aspiration pneumonia is prevented.
  2 Pressure sore healing is enhanced.
  3 Improves functional status.
  4 Provides comfort.
  5 Prolongs life.

Colonoscopy

- Indications common in the elderly.
- Safe if care taken with preparation and sedation, especially in those aged over 80 years of age.
- Complete examination rates may be reduced to between 50% and 60% in the very elderly.
- Abnormalities are common in the over-80s at about 80%. Diverticular disease is most common but also 11% show carcinoma, 25% polyps and 13% had multiple pathology.
- Both diagnostic and therapeutic potential, e.g. polypectomy and stent insertion.

Jaundice

- Surgical causes are common and must be identified rapidly before the condition becomes irremediable; ultrasound examination is the investigation of first choice.
- Medical causes of jaundice should be investigated and treated as in younger patients.
- Primary biliary cirrhosis and chronic hepatitis are more common in elderly patients than appreciated. Although occult, their prognosis in late life is often better than in younger patients.

Chronic liver disease

- All forms of chronic liver disease are increasing.
- Most have a prolonged course or 20–30 years leading to cirrhosis, 10 years with cirrhotic changes and an additional 5 years of severe symptoms in the period prior to death.
- Many patients are detected during this 30–40 year asymptomatic period as chance abnormalities on 'routine' liver-function tests – usually in middle-aged or elderly people.

- Such abnormalities if persistent or progressive need to be further investigated.
- The main types to be defined are;
  1 Alcoholic.
  2 Non-alcoholic fatty liver disease (NAFLD).
  3 Viral hepatitis – mainly B and C.
  4 Autoimmune hepatitis – primary biliary cirrhosis (PBC).
- Differential diagnosis is essential;
  1 Alcoholic damage identified by history. Men more commonly affected than women, but rate increasing in women.
  2 NAFLD – part of metabolic syndrome associated with raised blood pressure, obesity and insulin resistance. Men more affected than women.
  3 Viral hepatitis needs viral antibody titres. Hepatitis C most significant, found in reformed drug users, blood and blood product recipients prior to 1991. More common in Asians and sub-Saharians.
  4 PBC – autoimmune antibodies. More common in women than men.
- Liver biopsy may help confirm diagnosis and assist in monitoring progression.

- Differentiation important because of treatment options, e.g. antivirals, immuno-suppression, transplantation, lifestyle advice.

GI malignancy

Oesophagus

See p.106.

Gastric carcinoma

Although declining in incidence, it is still quite common; the rate for men is about twice that for women. The peak incidence is in the eight decade (see Figure 11.1) and most patients have advanced disease at diagnosis; it is therefore important to investigate late-onset dyspepsia. There is a genetic predisposition and an association with blood group A, atrophic gastritis and infection with *H. pylori*. Also there is considerable geographical variation in incidence and prognosis. It is particularly prevalent in Japan but the outlook for the disease there is more favourable; earlier diagnosis, which 'improves' survival time, may account for

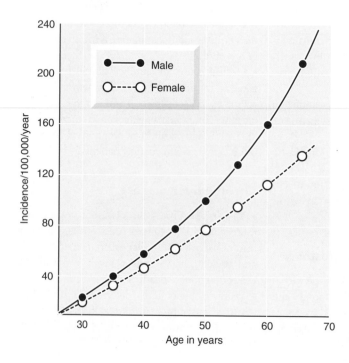

Figure 11.1 Carcinoma of the stomach. Special-risk groups are as follows: (i) old age (six times more common than in middle age); (ii) patients with pernicious anaemia (three to four times increased risk); (iii) previous gastric resection (five times as much risk); and (iv) patients with atrophic gastritis.

some of this but other factors are probably operating as well. Prolonged use of proton pump inhibitors may expose the patient to the risk of developing malignant change.

Clinically, indigestion, weight loss, vomiting, haematemesis, melaena and abdominal pain may occur. The diagnosis is confirmed by endoscopy or barium meal, and spread can be assessed by ultrasound or CT. The prognosis is poor and the treatment usually palliative; it may include gastrectomy, with adjuvant chemotherapy and radiotherapy or a bypass procedure.

Carcinoma of the pancreas

The incidence of pancreatic cancer is increasing in most developed countries although paradoxically not in Japan. It affects especially elderly men. Aetiological factors include cigarette smoking, high dietary fat and occupational exposure in the chemical and metal industries. The cancer is almost always far advanced at diagnosis and the prognosis is grim. Weight loss is usually striking and there may or may not be abdominal pain.

An ultrasound scan is a good initial investigation but CT is better able to define the extent of the growth. In most cases, the head of the pancreas is involved, leading to obstructive jaundice. Radical surgery is usually not an option, but stenting procedures provide relief from the symptoms of biliary obstruction.

Carcinoma of the colon and rectum

Colorectal cancer is the most common malignancy of the GI tract and the second most common cause of death from cancer in the UK; it is rare in Africa and Asia. This adenocarcinoma has a much lower grade of malignancy than gastric or pancreatic cancer; yet the 5-year survival of newly diagnosed cases is less than 30%. Patients with Crohn's disease and more especially those with polyposis and chronic ulcerative colitis are at increased risk of developing colorectal cancer (see also following box).

The clinical presentation is often rather vague, but malaise, abdominal pain and change of bowel habit, rectal bleeding, tenesmus or faecal

> ### Risk factors for carcinoma of the colon
>
> High red meat and animal fat intake.
> Low fibre intake from fruit and vegetables.
> Low physical activity.
> Obesity.
> Genetic tendency.
>
> *Note*: Hormone replacement therapy may be protective.

incontinence, depending on the site of the lesion, are the usual pointers. Up to 29% present as obstruction – they have a poor prognosis – with less than 20% having a 5-year survival and 40% have secondaries at the time of presentation. The diagnosis is confirmed by rectal examination and sigmoidoscopy, followed by abdominal CT and/or colonscopy or barium enema.

Treatment is surgical resection, ideally by a specialist colorectal surgeon. The use of self-expanding intraluminal stents looks promising, especially in obstructive cases of carcinoma of the colon.

The possibility of screening programmes, based on occult-blood detection and other techniques, is currently being pursued (see Table 11.2).

Clinical nutrition

The importance of food in the maintenance and recovery of health is once again being recognized. The connection between nutrition and health was more obvious to past practitioners. The current obsession with high-tech medicine has deflected our attention away from such simple but important factors in health care.

General nutritional standards in elderly people in the UK

The majority of elderly people living in their own homes within the UK enjoy a reasonable diet. Their standards and practices are likely to be higher than younger members of our society. Elderly people (even old men) usually know how to cook and take a reasonably varied and balanced diet maintaining the good habits of their earlier lives.

Table 11.2 Screening for carcinoma of the colon.

Faecal occult blood	Test annually or bi-annually
	Detects about 70% of cases
	False positives lead to anxiety and unnecessary investigations
Flexible sigmoidoscopy	Well tolerated
	Detects about 80% of cases
Barium enema	Safe but requires good bowel preparation and may miss small lesions
Colonoscopy	In expert hands, detects almost 100% of cases
	Expensive
	Requires bowel preparation
	Has risk of complications including perforation, bleeding + infection

The 1997/98 National Survey of Elderly People in the UK gave reassuring results. However, compared with the survey 30 years previously, the Medical Research Council found that people were eating less (energy intake was down 15%) but were increasing in weight. In 1997/98, 66% were considered overweight and only 5% underweight. The fat content of the diet was only slightly over the recommended levels but sugar was 7% above recommendations at 18%. All but up to 8% were taking sufficient vitamins and minerals; however, blood levels for folate, iron and vitamin C were subnormal in 10–15%. The adoption of a modified Mediterranean diet in a large cohort has demonstrated improved survival rates in participants of the EPIC study.

Factors which impair dietary intake

- Illness – the most common and most serious.
- Poor dental state – restricts dietary choice.
- Poverty.
- Being male.
- Living in the North, especially Scotland.
- Being in an institution.

Percentage of elderly people regularly taking common foods

- Potatoes and bread: 70%.
- Cooked vegetables: 66%.
- Salads, raw vegetables and fruit: 50%.
- Nutritional supplements: 30%.

Subnutrition

In the UK subnutrition is rarely due to poverty; it is more likely to be a consequence of eccentricity, illness or loneliness. Overnutrition, with excess of carbohydrate, fat and calories, is of greater frequency than malnutrition and these excesses are often associated with a deficient amount of dietary fibre. Displacement of nutrients by alcohol abuse is another significant cause for dietary distortion. Other important factors related to diet in old age are as follows:

- The incidence of subnutrition is difficult to determine as dietary assessment by recall (of foods eaten) or weighed surveys are unreliable in many elderly subjects and particularly in the most vulnerable.
- There is considerable doubt about the accuracy of recommended intakes – elderly people may need more or less than some other groups.
- Surveys in the UK indicated levels of malnutrition of about 3–7%.
- Poor diets may be either the result or the cause of declining health.
- Other factors are social isolation and bereavement.
- Low blood levels of vitamins, etc. are common in old age, especially in the frail elderly, but their significance is uncertain (Table 11.3).
- Hyperhomocysteinaemia is associated with low folate and vitamin B12 levels and increased rates of vascular disease and thromboembolism.

Causes of nutritional deficiency

1 Inability to shop or to prepare food, e.g. in cases of dementia, depression, poverty, loneliness, eccentricity, blindness or immobility due to arthritis or neurological disease.
2 Impaired appetite which may be part of the clinical picture of general malaise, may be due to biochemical abnormalities, be a consequence of the side-effects of drugs or indicate underlying GI disease.
3 Malabsorption.

Assessment of nutritional status in old age

This is a very difficult task but the following criteria have been found to be of value in some instances (all have drawbacks):
• Dietary history.
• Weight change.
• Height change.
• Skinfold thickness.
• Muscle power.
• Blood levels of nutrients.
• Clinical evidence of nutritional disease.
• BMI under 15 (twice demispan may be substituted for height).
• The Mini-Nutritional Assessment (MNA) combines measurements and answers to questions (see Table 11.3).
• Taken in isolation most of these abnormalities have multiple causes. A diagnosis of malnutrition can only be made if several abnormalities are

A simple recipe for a good diet

• Eat wholemeal bread not white bread.
• Have two portions of fresh vegetables daily.
• Eat three items of fresh fruit each day.
• Use 1/2 L (1 pint) of semi-skimmed milk daily, for drinking and for use in cooking.
• Have one egg per day.
• Have one portion of meat or fish per day (preferably oily fish).
• Drink at least 2 L of fluid a day.

Table 11.3 Incidence of low blood levels of vitamins, and so on. that have been reported in elderly subjects.

Subnutrition	Incidence
Haemoglobin <12 g	Up to 40% in institutions 6–9% elderly at home
Serum iron	Approximately 20%
Red cell folate	Approximately 20%
Serum B_{12}	Approximately 20%
Red cell B_6	Approximately 6%
Vitamin C	Up to 50%
Vitamin D	Up to 70%

Note: Wide variation due to different groups studied and methods used – all incidences of low levels are more common than actual evidence of clinical deficiencies.

found – the cause of the malnutrition must then be explored and, if possible, corrected.

Dietary deficiencies in old age

1 The most obvious are calories, protein and fluid.
2 Vitamin B group – refractory heart failure, macrocytic anaemia due to folate deficiency, also peripheral neuropathy, dementia, vascular disease and thromboembolism.
3 Vitamin C – scurvy.
4 Vitamin D – osteomalacia.
5 Vitamin E.
6 Zinc – especially from animal protein. Affects morbidity including macular degeneration.
7 Iron, calcium and selenium.
8 Fibre – diseases of 'Western civilization'.
Note: The routine use of vitamins and mineral supplements has not been proven in 'free range' elderly subjects. Justification for their use in vulnerable groups (the ill and the institutionalized) is more robust. Clearly, whenever deficiencies are identified, they should be corrected in all subjects.

Treatment of subnutrition in the community

1 Improve general health – treat underlying conditions.

2 Supplement intake – meals on wheels, luncheon clubs, meal preparation by home help, give vitamin supplements and high-calorie liquid diets.
3 Education of patients and carers.

Treatment of subnutrition in institutions

Up to 50% of elderly people admitted to hospital are under nourished. Many deteriorate further during their stay due to inappropriate foods and catering arrangements. The consequences are serious and lead to prolonged hospital stays due to:
1 Poor healing and recovery.
2 Increased risk of complications, e.g. infection and depression.
Attention needs to be paid at all times to:
1 Suitable foods, e.g. familiar, easy to swallow, enjoyable and energy rich.
2 Small and frequent feeds – not large, widely spaced boluses.
3 Assistance with feeding when necessary, e.g. food placed within reach, modified utensils, cutting up of food and encouragement from staff.
4 Eating in selected groups at a table increases both pleasure and intake.
5 Artificial feeding when appropriate – see Chapter 16.
NB: Please note, these measures should also apply to catering arrangements in care homes.

Obesity/overnutrition

The epidemic of morbid obesity, which is currently affecting the USA, is heading towards Europe. Although cases do occur in old people, in the UK they remain rare. Generally such people remain well whilst living within their limits. However, disaster is likely to strike at the first significant change in health status.

The period of enforced restriction influenced by illness will lead to the rapid loss of strength. After just a few days it may become impossible for them to remobilize independently.

In addition their vast bulk will hinder attempts at assistance by care workers. Health and safety regulations will insist that hoists are used and will therefore complicate any attempts at rehabilitation. These patients may (unkindly) be compared to beached whales – if not quickly refloated, they are doomed.

The extra nutritional reserves they carry may be of benefit. However, their large size will exaggerate the complications of immobility, especially hypostatic pneumonia and pressure sores. The latter are likely to develop in deep tissue between pressure points and only become obvious when the deep abscess suddenly discharges through the skin to reveal a deep necrotic cavity below.

To carry any excess weight into old age is detrimental to wellbeing through the worsening of any one or more of the following:
1 Angina.
2 Breathlessness.
3 Poor glucose control.
4 Poor blood pressure control.
5 Destruction of weight-bearing joints.
6 Depression and loss of self-esteem.
7 Peri-operative complications.
8 Delayed rehabilitation.

At retirement, all overweight subjects should be encouraged to take changes in lifestyle seriously and make every effort to improve their ways.

In cases of sudden and unexplained weight gain it is important to exclude endocrine causes (e.g. myxoedema) or fluid retention, such as occurs in heart failure.

Further information

Borum M.L. (ed.) (1999) *Clinics in Geriatric Medicine*, Vol. 15.3, *Gastroenterology*. W.B. Saunders.

Gelb A.M. (ed.) (1996) *Clinical Gastroenterology in the Elderly*. Dekker.

Thomas, D. (ed.) (2002) *Clinics in Geriatric Medicine*, Vol. 18.4, *Undernutrition in Older Adults*. W.B. Saunders.

Chapter 12

Disorders of homeostasis and metabolism

Age changes

There is a reduction in lean body mass and body water and usually a relative increase in fat (Figure 12.1).

Endocrine changes

Some elderly people have unmeasurably low levels of growth hormone; in some, it fails to respond to an insulin tolerance test. Some male subjects have global muscle wasting, and the administration of human growth hormone has been shown to increase lean body mass and reduce adipose tissue but without clear benefit to quality of life.

Other hormonal changes include:

- Serum noradrenaline ↑ (but β-receptors ↓).
- Insulin ↑ (due to insulin resistance): carbohydrate tolerance diminishes.

- Arginine vasopressin (AVP) ↓ susceptibility to hyponatraemia ↑.
- Atrial natriuretic peptide ↑ and nocturia ↑.
- Oestrogen and progesterone in women ↓, follicle stimulating hormone (FSH) and luteinising hormone (LH) ↑.
- Testosterone in men ↓, FSH and LH ↑.
- Renin and aldosterone ↓.

Adenomas are common in anterior pituitary, thyroid and adrenal glands.

Fluid and electrolyte imbalance

Acutely unwell elderly patients are very often fluid-depleted or fluid-overloaded, and occasionally both.

Reasons for vulnerability to dehydration:

1 Reduction in body water.
2 Inadequate intake due to:
  (a) Impaired thirst response.

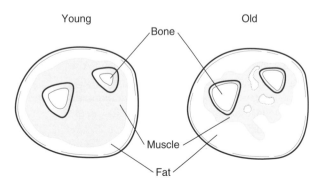

Figure 12.1 Diagramatic cross-section through a young and an old leg to show change in composition.

(b) Dementia or depression.

(c) Immobility.

(d) Reluctance through fear of being 'caught short'.

(e) Swallowing difficulty.

(f) Acute illness.

(mainly affects intracellular compartment, with thirst, confusion and drowsiness)

3 Loss:

(a) Reduced concentrating ability by kidney.

(b) Diuretics.

(c) Diabetes, diarrhoea and vomiting.

Loss of salt and water often replaced by water, tea, and so on. Mixed salt and water depletion presents with confusion, weakness, loss of tissue, turgor, tachycardia and postural hypotension, as extracellular compartment is mainly affected.

Hyponatraemia

This is common in frail old patients and is due to too little sodium, too much water or both. Do not treat the sodium level in isolation. Decide whether the patient is dehydrated, euvolaemic or fluid overloaded.

If the patient is dry, salt and water have been lost either through the kidneys (diuretics especially thiazides, renal failure, osmotic diuresis), the gut (vomiting, diarrhoea, fistula, adenoma) or skin (burns).

If the patient is oedematous, there is relative water excess due to fluid retention (in cardiac failure, liver failure or nephrotic syndrome) or excess water intake (usually overenthusiastic dextrose after surgery).

If the patient does not appear dry or wet, one of the preceding may be developing. However, if the urine is concentrated (sodium >20 mmol/L in the presence of hyponatraemia) and the plasma is dilute with a low plasma osmolality (<260 mmol/kg), the syndrome of inappropriate antidiuretic hormone (SIADH) is present. This leads to intracellular water accumulation in the brain with confusion, headache, lethargy, coma and fits.

Causes of SIADH

- Drugs, especially SSRIs, venlafaxine, opiates, certain sulphonylureas.
- Malignancy.
- CNS, e.g. stroke.
- Chest disease, e.g. pneumonia.

Treatment

- Underlying cause.
- Water restriction/intravenous infusion of normal saline as appropriate.
- Demeclocycline (blocks action of ADH on tubule).

Hypernatraemia

This is usually due to water loss in excess of sodium loss and occurs where patients are unable to take in enough water to meet their needs.

Oedema

If oedema is present to or below the knee of a patient in a chair, slip a hand under the thigh and, if oedema is present there too, lean the patient forward to check for a sacral pad. Not all oedema is heart failure.

Some causes of ankle oedema

Raised venous pressure:
- Gravity (prolonged sitting).
- Cardiac failure.
- Pelvic mass.

The following causes are often unilateral:
- Venous insufficiency (side of hip surgery).
- DVT.
- Lack of muscle pump (side of hemiparesis).
- Over-active muscle pump in one leg (tremor in Parkinson's disease) makes bilateral oedema appear unilateral.

Fluid retention:
- Cardiac failure.
- Drugs [(NSAID), steroids, calcium channel blockers, glitazones].
- Renal failure.

Hypoalbuminaemia

• Nutritional, hepatic disease or protein loss via kidney, bowels or extensive skin loss (dip-stick urine for protein).

Lymphatic obstruction

• Usually malignant.

Inflammatory

• Localized.

Hypokalaemia

Another common finding in geriatric practice, often due to diuretics or GI loss (remember the laxative abuser), exacerbated by inadequate dietary intake (many patients have diets deficient in fruit, vegetables and meat). Mild Conn's syndrome is probably under recognized. It has been reported that sick elderly females, in particular, may develop 'acute transient hypokalaemia', probably due to a shift into the cells, which usually self-corrects within a few days. Hypokalaemia exacerbates digoxin toxicity. Replace orally or by slow intravenous infusion if severe. If the response is poor, check for low magnesium, as correcting this helps.

Hyperkalaemia

This occurs in renal failure and rhabdomyolysis (both of which may follow a collapse and long lie). However, drugs are the common culprits. In old age, cardiac failure can often be managed with frusemide rather than the potassium retaining combination of frusemide and amiloride that is often needed in middle age. A combination of an ACE inhibitor and spironolactone may be evidence-based treatment for cardiac failure in drug trials but, particularly if Frumil® is also prescribed, will usually result in dangerous hyperkalaemia with older kidneys! Give intravenous calcium, insulin and glucose and calcium resonium. Doses of ACE inhibitor and potassium-sparing diuretic that control heart failure

when the patient is well, result in hypokalaemia and renal failure in an intercurrent illness with dehydration. On admission, consider holding the next dose of such drugs until the urea, creatinine and electrolytes are available.

Diabetes mellitus

Definition

The WHO (1999) (see NICE guidelines) advises that the ranges of blood glucose indicative of diabetes mellitus are as follows:
• Random venous plasma glucose ≥ 11.1 mmol/L or
• Fasting plasma glucose ≥ 7.0 mmol/L or
• Plasma glucose ≥ 11.1 mmol/L at 2 hr after a 75-g oral glucose load (oral glucose tolerance test).

Epidemiology

Prevalence rises with age up to the highest age band studied (84 years) and is higher in Afro-Caribbean and Asian people than white people in the UK. It is estimated that 1.4 million people in the UK have diabetes, 80% of whom have Type 2 diabetes. Because of the ageing population and increase in obesity, this is predicted to rise to 3 million by 2010. Half the diabetic population and a quarter of insulin users are elderly. A common 'ballpark' figure is that 5% of people aged 70 have known diabetes and the same number have unrecognized impaired glucose tolerance.

Mechanism

The impairment of glucose tolerance in old age is mainly caused by reduced tissue sensitivity to insulin at post-receptor level. There is also β-cell dysfunction; the pancreas is less able to secrete insulin in response to a glucose load and the rapid post-prandial spike of secretion is lost. The older diabetic usually has Type 2 diabetes, although the number of Type 1 graduates to old age will increase steadily. Occasionally, Type 1 diabetes occurs *de novo* in an older person.

Effects

Diabetics aged 65–75 have twice the cardiovascular and all-cause mortality – but thereafter it tends to revert towards normal. One-third has visual impairment, more often due to cataract than to retinopathy, and the amputation rate is enormously increased and cognitive and psychosocial function is generally impaired. A common end stage comprises poor cardiac function, renal failure and marked oedema.

Management

Management of the diabetes must be part of a holistic approach to cardiovascular risk and will depend greatly on the circumstances of the patient; a frail nursing home resident requires different care to an otherwise fit and independent 75-year-old who should attend a diabetic clinic.

Aims include a feeling of well-being and the avoidance of hypoglycaemia, which can cause brain damage or injury, but tight enough control is required to avoid complications in younger elderly patients. Haemoglobin A1C (HbA1C) should be measured at 2- to 6-monthly intervals. Dietary advice concentrates on weight reduction in the obese, reducing fat intake and ensuring that carbohydrates are of a high-fibre, unrefined, polysaccharide type. Because of the failure of the post-prandial insulin spike, the concept of the glycaemic index of food may be particularly useful. Carbohydrates vary greatly with regard to how rapidly they increase blood sugar. Some are absorbed quickly and blood glucose levels increase very rapidly ('high GI' foods), while others release glucose slowly and have little effect ('low GI' foods). Carbohydrates are ranked on a scale of 1 – 100 with glucose being used as the reference point of 100. Regular exercise is highly beneficial. Rimonabant, a cannabinoid CB 1 receptor antagonist, could be useful helping weight loss. Smoking must be discouraged, and statins prescribed for hypercholesterolaemia (at least up to 80 years) and hypertension treated vigorously if the patient can tolerate this. ACE inhibitors or ARBs have a particular role in reducing microscopic albuminuria.

Patients require basic education about diabetes and how lifestyle changes will help if they are to adhere to their diet. Periodic surveillance, including eyes and feet, is at least as important as in younger subjects.

If drugs are necessary, the best data come from the United Kingdom Prospective Diabetes Study (UKPDS). Metformin, which decreases gluconeogenesis and increases peripheral utilization of glucose, is first-line, whereas it used to be restricted to obese patients. Care must be taken if there is renal impairment (contraindicated if creatinine > 130 μmol/L) or risk of sudden renal deterioration. Sulphonylureas, which augment insulin secretion, are another option: those with short half-lives (e.g. glipizide 3–6 h) are favoured (avoid chlorpropramide and glibenclamide). Weight gain may be a problem. Glimepramide is a sulphonylurea marketed as a post-prandial glucose regulator. The α-glucosidase inhibitor acarbose, which delays starch absorption, is often not well tolerated because of flatulence. Newer drugs include repaglinide, a metiglinide and nateglinide, the first of a new group of glucose-responsive amino acid derivatives, which are both short-acting and restore early phase insulin secretion and reduce post-prandial glucose spikes. They may be useful in the elderly as there is little risk of hypoglycaemia. The thiazolidinedione derivatives ('glitazones') activate the peroxisome-proliferator-activated receptor gamma (PPARγ) in the cell nucleus. The normal ligand is free fatty acids. Gene transcription is altered resulting in increased glucose uptake and utilization in the periphery. Thiazolidinediones sensitize adipose tissue, liver, and muscle to insulin. However, they are not recommended in heart failure, a common problem in the elderly diabetic; so experience is limited. New drugs include vildagliptin, which increases the levels of glucagon-like peptide (GLP-1) by inhibiting dipeptidyl peptidase-4, the enzyme that inactivates GLP-1. Vildagliptin is one of several incretin enhancer drugs in development; incretins increase secretion of insulin from the pancreas as blood glucose levels rise after a meal. Another drug, exanetide mimics GLP-1, but has to be given subcutaneously. Whatever drug is chosen, further education is essential to make sure the patient understands how and when to take the drug, and how to manage hypoglycaemia.

If control is poor, it is a mistake to be too reluctant to institute insulin, which makes the poorly controlled diabetic feel vastly better. However, the common twice-daily injection regime (of, e.g., Mixtard®) can pose practical difficulties in those living alone whose intellect, vision or dexterity is too limited to permit self-injection. A single daily injection of Glargine® can achieve adequate control with minimal risk of hypoglycaemia. Combinations of insulin and tablets are increasing used. Foot care and regular chiropody are particularly important in the elderly diabetic.

Hyperosmolar crisis

Diabetic crises and complications do not present any special features in old people apart from hyperosmolar coma. This typically occurs in patients with Type 2 diabetes that has often hitherto caused very little problem. An osmotic diuresis leads to insidiously progressive dehydration and hypotension, culminating in stupor or coma. However, because there is still some endogenous insulin, the body does not switch to metabolic pathways resulting in ketone production. Extreme hyperglycaemia, hypernatraemia and uraemia are typical. The aim here is steady correction of the metabolic derangement. Avoid doing things too rapidly and remember rehydration is more important than insulin. It is safest to give normal saline, as this will be relatively dilute in comparison with the plasma. Depending on the severity and the patient's cardiac status, give a litre over 1–2 h and assess the effect. Continue with a litre over 2, 4, 6 h, and so on. It may be necessary to give 10 L of fluid over and above output over the first 48 h or so, ideally monitored by the central venous pressure (CVP) line. Wait an hour before giving any insulin, the glucose often falls dramatically with rehydration, but if it is needed 1 unit per hour would be a typical dose. The risk of venous thrombosis is high so give a full preventative dose of heparin (e.g. 40 mg Clexane®). Those who survive do not need insulin unless control remains poor.

Thyroid disease – function tests

Normal function is usually preserved until at least 80 years of age but in centenarians TSH and free T3 levels may decline. In the seriously ill patient, the TSH, T3 and T4 levels may all be misleadingly low ('sick euthyroid syndrome'), and amiodarone and anticonvulsants often interfere with thyroid-function tests (TFTs). Always check TFTs before starting amiodarone and remember that this will interfere with radioiodine treatment. Both hypo- and hyperthyroidism are difficult to diagnose clinically in old age and many geriatricians routinely check TSH in any significant illness.

Hyperthyroidism

Presentation is atypical – AF, heart failure, weight loss, proximal myopathy, functional decline. The thyroid may be nodular or impalpable – sometimes retrosternal. Treatment is carbimazole and a beta-blocker if the heart rate is high, prior to definitive therapy with I^{131}. Carbimazole can be given in a dose aiming for normal thyroid hormone level or in a dose to block all production with thyroxine replacement (see BNF). Remember to give written advice about sore throat on carbimazole (neutropaenia). The management of amiodarone-induced thyrotoxicosis is controversial. Some advocate ignoring a raised free T_4 but treating raised T_3 with carbimazole and steroids.

Hypothyroidism

Hypothyroidism affects 5% of people aged over 60 and it may be due to Hashimoto's disease, I^{131} treatment, surgery, idiopathic or, occasionally, secondary to pituitary failure. Clinical pointers include impaired cognition and slow-relaxing ankle jerks. Treatment is with thyroxine 25 µg, with similar increments every 3–4 weeks until on a daily dose of around 100 µg, the patient feels well and the TSH confirms euthyroidism. If a profoundly hypothyroid woman is admitted and 100 µg thyroxine tablets are brought in with her, do not just write them on the chart – it is very likely she has not been taking them. Get advice and if in doubt build up from a low dose to avoid precipitating an MI.

Adrenal disease

Cushing's syndrome

The commonest cause in old age is iatrogenic. Older people are often left on higher doses of steroid than they need, particularly for polymyalgia rheumatica, which usually burns itself out after a couple of years. Older people on steroids are particularly prone to fluid retention, heart failure, diabetes, proximal myopathy and osteoporosis (always give bone protection) and high doses may lead to acute confusion, 'steroid psychosis'.

Addison's disease

Adrenal insufficiency may occur acutely, usually when there is an acute severe illness in a patient with iatrogenic adrenal suppression due to long-term steroid treatment. Chronic adrenal insufficiency is due to adrenal destruction, e.g. TB or metastases and not surprisingly (since the presentation is insidious even in middle age) has to be thought about in order to carry out a short synacthen test.

Autonomic nervous system

The autonomic nervous system (ANS) is the part of the nervous system most closely involved in homoeostatic mechanisms. There is some age-related decline in function and more obvious problems result from central or peripheral neurological damage, e.g. diabetes, alcoholism, Parkinson's disease (less common but more severe – multisystem atrophy), uraemia, drug-induced neuropathies, amyloidosis, autoimmune disorders and paraneoplastic syndromes. Common manifestations are orthostatic hypotension, erectile dysfunction, impaired bladder emptying, gastric paresis,

---

Accidental hypothermia: a salutary tale

One day, the neighbours notice that an old lady who lives by herself has not taken the milk in or drawn back the curtains and there is no sign of life from her house. They have a key, so they let themselves in and, after shouting for her with no response, they eventually find her in her bedroom, on the floor, in a dazed condition, wearing only her nightdress. Hesitant to move her, they call the GP and together they manage to get her into bed.

The GP notices that the room is cold – there is no heating and there is a window open. The GP checks that there is no obvious injury from the fall, such as a fractured neck of femur, that there is no obvious illness which may have caused her to fall, such as a hemiplegia, and assumes she may have had some debilitating illness, e.g. pneumonia, that made her collapse on the floor as she tried to get out of bed to visit the toilet. She is drowsy, croaky of voice, very slow of movement and response, and her limbs are strikingly rigid. The GP puts a hand on her abdomen and finds that it feels unnaturally cool. Her pulse rate is 50 b.p.m., her BP 100/70 and the tympanic thermometer reveals a core temperature of 31°C. **Why?**

- It has been a cold March night.
- She has a serious illness – pneumonia (drugs such as alcohol and phenothiazines also predispose to hypothermia).
- She is only wearing a nightdress and has spent most of the night on the floor.
- Her ability to detect a falling ambient temperature is less than that of a young person. The previous evening, she forgot to put on the woolly nightcap her thoughtful neighbour gave her for Christmas, not realizing that 40% of the body's heat is lost through the scalp. She also failed to close the window and to plug in the fan heater that her daughter had bought her. She has never had central heating installed.
- As her body temperature started to fall, her ANS failed to cut down heat loss by cutaneous vasoconstriction and failed to increase heat production by shivering.

The three main factors that have combined to produce this typical clinical picture are: systemic illness, exposure to cold and ANS dysfunction; if sufficiently severe, only one of these factors need be present to cause accidental hypothermia (core temperature less than 35°C).

diarrhoea or constipation. A battery of tests for autonomic function is described in the paper (Allan, 2006).

Accidental hypothemia

Clinical features

Above 32°C the features may be those of an under-lying disease or of functional decline. Below 32°C the features are as described for the aforemen-tioned patient and, below 27°C, 75% of the patients are comatose. Pancreatitis, hypoglycaemia and ventricular arrhythmias are among the complica-tions. Everyone seems to remember the J waves (at the R-ST junction or 'J point'), but you diagnose hypothermia with a low reading thermometer, not an ECG. Over 30°C the mortality is about 33%, but below 30°C it approaches 70%.

Management

At a core temperature just below 35°C, it is reason-able to re-warm the patient at home and counsel (scold) to prevent recurrence. More serious cases (30–34°C) have traditionally received gradual pas-sive re-warming in hospital at 0.5–1.0°C per hour to avoid sudden profound hypotension. Avoid instrumentation, which may precipitate serious arrhythmia. Below 30°C some would argue that conservative measures constitute losing tactics and that admission to the ITU is required for active re-warming, using a 'Bair hugger' or forced-air warming system. However, most elderly patients have to take their chance on an open ward.

Other dangers of extreme weather

Cold kills in other ways, and in an average winter there are 40,000 deaths in England and Wales above the expected number, mainly due to vascu-lar causes. Platelets, haematocrit, blood viscosity, plasma cholesterol and, in old men at least, systolic BP tends to rise on exposure to the cold. Blood fibrinogen levels may rise during the winter months. Slipping on icy pavements is a further hazard. The incidence of strokes and the mortality rate also tend to rise among elderly people in the UK during heat waves. Food poisoning is another hazard of heat waves.

Further information

Allan, L.M., Ballard, C.G., Allen, J., Murray, A., Davidson, A.W., McKeith, I.G., *et al.* (2006) Auto-nomic dysfunction in dementia, Dec. 18; [Epub ahead of print] http://jnnp.bmj.com/cgi/rapid-pdf/jnnp. 2006.102343v1

British Medical Journal home page; type diabetes in search: http://www.bmj.com/

Curry, R.W. and Wilson, G.R.. (2005) Subclinical thyroid disease. *American Family of Physician,* **72,** 1517–24. http://www.aafp.org/afp/20051015/1517.html

Diabetes UK (formerly the British Diabetic Associa-tion) website has lots of information for patients, carers and professionals: http://www.diabetes.org.uk/ (use the search facility to check diagnostic criteria, the latest on the NSF, etc.)

Heine, R.J., Diamant, M., Mbanya, J.-C. and Nathan, D.M. (2006) Management of hypergly-caemia in type 2 diabetes: the end of recurrent failure? *British Medical Journal,* **333,** 1200–4, doi:10.1136/bmj.39022.462546.80 http://www.bmj.com/cgi/content/full/333/7580/1200

J wave: http://www.monroecc.edu/depts/pstc/backup/parcm10a.htm

Minniti, G., Esposito, V., Piccirilli, M., Fratticci, A., Santoro A. and Jaffrain-Rea M.L. (2005) Diagnosis and management of pituitary tumours in the elderly: a review based on personal experience and evidence of literature. *European Journal of Endocrinology,* **153,** 723–35.

NICE guidelines for the management of diabetes September 2002: http://www.nice.org.uk/ and search for diabetes)

Pimenta, E. and Calhoun, D.A. (2006) Primary aldosteronism: diagnosis and treatment. *Journal of Clinical Hypertension,* **8,** 887–93.

Reynolds, R.M., Padfield, P.L. and Seckl, J.R. (2006) Disorders of sodium balance. *British Medical Jour-nal,* **332,** 702–5.

Scottish intercollegiate guidelines website – this is a super website with a wide range of material. The diabetes guidelines do not specifically cover the elderly but feet are well dealt with! http://www.sign.ac.uk

United Kingdom Department of Health website with press releases explaining latest policies. Relevant examples here include 'Keep warm, keep well': http://www.doh.gov.uk

Yeates, K.E., Singer, M. and Ross Morton A. (2004) Salt and water: a simple approach to hyponatremia. *Canadian Medical Association Journal*, **170**, 365–9. http://www.cmaj.ca/cgi/content/full/170/3/365

Chapter 13

Genitourinary disease

Ageing changes

1 In old age, renal function is reduced to about 50% of the peak (i.e. that achieved aged 30).

2 Serum urea in healthy old age remains normal in spite of falling renal function.

3 Creatinine reflects muscle bulk; so beware the frail elderly patient with a 'normal' creatinine.

4 The estimated glomerular filtration rate (eGFR) can be calculated using the creatinine, gender and age.

5 The ageing kidney has impaired ability both to concentrate urine and to process an extra water load quickly. This is one explanation for the increased incidence of nocturia in old age. The ability to concentrate urine falls from 1300 to 850 mOsm/L.

6 There is loss of renal mass, affecting the cortex more than the medulla in 46% of the 'normal' elderly kidneys.

7 Reduced renal function is due to:
- Loss of number of glomeruli combined with increased percentage of sclerosed glomeruli; and
- Reduced renal blood flow, again affecting the cortex more than the medulla.
- Poor response to ADH.

These effects are exaggerated in hypertension, diabetes or pyelonephritis in earlier life.

8 The combination of renal ageing changes and systemic or renal disease may lead to rapid and dramatic renal failure in elderly patients.

9 Atrophic changes, secondary to lower oestrogen levels, occur in the urogenital tract of post-menopausal women.

10 Prostatic size increases with age.

11 The incidence of unstable bladder increases with age. Detrusor instability is due to sudden uncontrollable surges in bladder pressure secondary to contractions whilst filling. This is associated with neurological degeneration.

Renal failure in old age

Pre-renal and post-renal causes are most frequently responsible for this presentation. Therefore, management includes:

- Assessing the patient's fluid status and rehydrating as appropriate.
- Excluding renal-tract obstruction by examination and ultrasound. Timely treatment of obstruction can return the renal function to normal.
- Excluding urinary-tract infection (UTI) by sending a midstream urine (MSU) sample.
- Intrinsic renal disease is not often of paramount clinical importance in geriatric patients, but all medications should be scrutinized to omit those that damage renal function further and to reduce the doses of those excreted by the kidney.
- Age alone should not be used as a contraindication for renal dialysis. In fact, many elderly patients adopt a very philosophical approach, which makes them very suitable – especially for continuous

ambulatory peritoneal dialysis (CAPD). Up to 20% of dialysis patients are aged over 70 years.

Intrinsic renal disease

1 Nephrotic syndrome. In a series of patients aged over 50 years with nephrotic syndrome (diabetics were excluded), the underlying cause in order of incidence was:
  (a) Membranous glomerulonephritis.
  (b) Proliferative glomerulonephritis.
  (c) Amyloid: usually secondary to long-standing inflammatory disease, e.g. bronchiectasis, osteo-myelitis or rheumatoid arthritis.
  (d) Minimal-change glomerulonephritis.
2 Diabetic nephropathy. No special features in old age.
3 Myeloma: see Chapter 14.
4 Nephrocalcinosis/stones. Exclude vitamin D intoxication, gout and hyperparathyroidism – all occur more frequently in old age.

Urinary-tract infection

• UTIs (bacteriuria greater than 10^5/mL) are common in old age.
• Twenty per cent of people over the age of 65 will experience UTI.
• This increases to 50% of women in institutional care.
• Female-to-male ratio: 3:1.
• Escherichia coli is the most common pathogen. Others include Proteus and Klebsiella.
• Asymptomatic bacteriuria with no pyuria does not require treatment.
• Pyelonephritis is responsible for 20% of the cases of renal failure.
  Precipitating factors for UTIs in old age are:
1 High incidence of urinary stasis:
  (a) Poor bladder emptying.
  (b) Lower urinary-tract syndrome secondary to prostatic hypertrophy.
  (c) Bladder diverticula.
2 Loss of cohesiveness of the female urethra due to reduced oestrogen.
3 Associated disorders:
  (a) Diabetes.

  (b) Atherosclerosis.
  (c) Immobility.
  (d) Indwelling catheter.
4 Urinary-tract stones.

Unusual presentations of UTI in old age

1 Acute confusional state – catheterization may be required to obtain specimen; alternatively organisms may be isolated from a blood culture.
2 New urinary incontinence.
3 Increasing drowsiness due to worsening renal failure.

Management

1 Culture organism from urine or blood.
2 Maintain good fluid input (greater than 2 L/day).
3 Give appropriate antibiotics (trimethoprim best 'blind treatment').
4 Reverse precipitating cause, if possible (see earlier).

Obstructive nephropathy

Obstructive nephropathy is secondary to a blockage anywhere along the urinary tract.

Lesion in urethra

1 Males (usually).
2 Past history of previous episodes of sexually transmitted disease.
3 Bladder palpable or demonstrable on ultrasound.
4 Catheterization is difficult or impossible, consider suprapubic approach and obtain expert help.

Bladder-neck obstruction

Prostate pathology

1 By the eighth decade, 50% of prostates contain areas of benign nodular hyperplasia, chronic prostatitis, and pre-malignant changes. The patient may complain of hesitancy, urgency, and nocturia and poor stream.
2 Fewer than half of all men with benign prostatic hypertrophy develop symptoms. In mild cases or

in patients who are a poor surgical risk, treatment with α-adrenoceptor antagonists (e.g. indoramin and doxazosin) may be beneficial. Newer, more selective alpha-blockers such as tamsulosin are said to be less likely to cause orthostatic hypotension.

3 Rectal examination first essential step in diagnosis – enlargement may be confirmed by rectal ultrasound.

4 Only 1% of prostatic cancers cause problems during life, but it is the second most frequent malignancy in men.

5 Any suspicious nodules should be biopsied to exclude carcinoma; this can be done transrectally.

6 Raised prostate-specific antigen (PSA) supports the diagnosis of carcinoma, especially if the ratio of free (unbound) PSA to total PSA is low. A very high PSA suggests metastatic disease.

7 Transurethral prostatectomy (TURP) is the treatment of choice for benign prostatic hypertrophy (BPH), but there is increasing anxiety about safety (blood loss and absorption of irrigation fluids) and need for repeat surgery in older patients.

8 Treatment of carcinoma (orchidectomy, hormone therapy, radical surgery or radiotherapy) depends on the spread of the disease and patient's preferences.

9 In the case of the chance finding of malignant cells in a TURP specimen, the management remains problematic and many patients will live trouble-free.

Gynaecological problems – detectable on pelvic examination

1 Malignancy of female genital tract and presence of fibroids.

2 Hormone-deficient changes in mucosa of trigone of bladder.

Spread of rectal malignancy

Detectable on rectal examination and on CT scanning.

Faecal impaction

Must always be excluded, as it is readily reversible.

Neurological disease

Affects bladder emptying.

Iatrogenic disease

Anticholinergic drugs such as tolterodine and oxybutynin are common precipitants.

Retroperitoneal disease

Malignancy and fibrosis (latter may be drug induced, e.g. by beta-blockers and methysergide). It is usually associated with a very high ESR.

Unilateral disease

Due to ureteric obstruction, secondary to stones, malignancy or fibrosis.

Drugs and the kidneys

1 Nephrotoxic drugs:
   (a) Antibiotics, e.g. gentamicin, vancomycin and tetracycline.
   (b) Analgesics, e.g. NSAIDs and phenacetin.
   (c) Disease-modifying anti-rheumatic drugs (DMARDs), e.g. penicillamine and gold.

2 Overdosage of drugs acting on kidneys, i.e. diuretics leading to dehydration, hypotension and electrolyte imbalance, to the extent of causing marked renal failure.

3 Renal changes causing drug toxicity, i.e. drugs excreted via the kidneys – best example is digoxin.

4 ACE inhibitors may precipitate renal failure if used in patients with silent renovascular disease.

Blood pressure and the kidneys

1 Renal disease may cause hypertension, e.g. chronic pyelonephritis.

2 The overtreatment of high blood pressure will impair renal function. Yet, untreated hypertension may result in renal failure!

3 About one-third of elderly patients with hypertension have impaired renal function.

4 Hypotension, e.g. after bleeding, myocardial infarction or pulmonary embolus, may result in renal shutdown and acute renal failure especially where renal function is already compromised by extreme old age or pathological changes.

5 Renal artery stenosis (RAS) may first present as a marked deterioration in renal function after treatment with an ACE inhibitor.

6 Bilateral renal artery stenosis can also present as 'flash' pulmonary oedema, which is thought be due to the combination of the RAS and fluid overload plus diastolic ventricular dysfunction.

Haematuria

See Table 13.1.

Urinary incontinence

Urinary incontinence is defined as 'the involuntary loss of urine sufficient in volume or frequency to be a social or a health problem'.

• It affects 50% of older people in hospital and nursing homes and 35% of those living in the community.

• It is often concealed by the patient because of embarrassment.

• Only 25% of the affected women consult a doctor.

• It is twice as common in women as in men. This is because of the female anatomy, and because low oestrogen levels lead to reduced cohesiveness of the urethra, making it patulous.

Complications

• Embarrassment leads to fear of going out and this leads to social isolation.

• Depression.

• Sexual problems.

• Huge burden on patients and their carers: financial (pads are expensive) and workload (extra washing).

• Increased risk of institutionalization.

• Skin irritation and maceration may lead to pressure sores (see pressure sores page 152).

Reversible causes

The mnemonic 'diapers' is helpful! See Table 13.2.

Table 13.1 Causes, investigations and management of haematuria.

Cause	Investigations	Management
Bleeding diathesis	Abnormal clotting, low platelets	Review need for anticoagulants, check liver function
UTI	MSU, blood cultures	Antibiotics, treat predisposing factors
Transitional cell carcinoma of the bladder	Cystoscopy	Transurethral resection of bladder tumour with regular review
Ureteric stones	IVU, ultrasound	Extracorporeal shockwave lithotripsy, endoscopic removal preventative measures
Benign prostatic hypertrophy	Clinical examination	Alpha-blockers, TURP
Carcinoma of the prostate	Biopsy, PSA	Treat as appropriate
Intrinsic renal disease	Consider renal biopsy if appropriate	Treat as appropriate
Renal cell carcinoma	Ultrasound or CT abdomen, urine cytology	Treat as appropriate
Contamination with vaginal blood	Obtain clean catch specimen, with catheter if necessary	See vaginal bleeding
Immune complex disease, e.g. bacterial endocarditis	Blood cultures, echocardiography, etc.	Treat underlying condition

Table 13.2 Reversible causes of urinary incontinence.

	Investigations	Management
Delirium	MSU, CXR, FBC, U & Es	Treat underlying cause
Infection	MSU	Treat infection
Atrophic urethritis		Topical oestrogen in females
Pharmaceuticals: sedatives, caffeine diuretics antidepressants, alcohol		Use alternatives if possible, try lower doses
Psychiatric: secondary to dementia, behavioural problems		Exclude treatable causes, toilet regularly
Excess urine production	Serum glucose, calcium	Treat diabetes, hypercalcaemia
Restricted mobility	Joint and neurological examination	Physiotherapy, walking aids, commode , disabled toilets
Stool impaction	Rectal examination	Regular laxatives, adequate fluid intake

Types of incontinence

1 Stress incontinence: involuntary leaking of urine when sneezing, coughing and exercising.
Most common in multi-parous women and those who have had pelvic surgery. In men the most common cause is sphincter damage after radical prostatectomy.

Non-surgical treatments: pelvic floor exercises remain the gold standard. They should be prescribed for the individual woman. The patient must be encouraged to continue with the exercises long-term, or the benefit is lost. Ring pessaries are useful for women with significant vaginal prolapse who are not fit for or do not wish to have surgery. Some women benefit from the use of duloxetine (a serotonin-noradrenalin reuptake inhibitor), which works at the level of the spinal cord increasing urethral sphincter tone, but nausea is a very common side effect.

Surgical procedures: there are now two non-invasive procedures available. Periurethral injection of collagen improves continence, but needs to be repeated every 2–3 years. Tension-free vaginal tape (TVT) can be used to raise the middle portion of the urethra and improve continence. It is done under local anaesthetic and as a day case. If this fails and the patient is fit enough, she can go on to have a colpo-suspension to elevate the bladder neck, or an anterior repair for prolapse.

2 Urge incontinence: is frequent and urgent passing of small amounts of urine, sometimes with so little warning that the patient does not reach the toilet in time. This is due to detrusor instability. It increases with age and is associated with hyper-reflexia in neurological conditions such as stroke, multiple sclerosis and Parkinson's disease.

Treatment: anti-muscarinic anticholinergic agents such as oxybutynin and tolterodine. Tolterodine is said to be more specific to the bladder muscarinic receptors and therefore cause less dry mouth and confusion. Trospium does not cross the blood–brain barrier and is therefore even less likely to cause confusion.

3 Mixed incontinence: is a combination of the symptoms of stress and urge incontinence, and is probably the most common presentation in older people.

4 Overflow incontinence: is most common in men with benign prostatic hypertrophy, but may also be secondary to prostatic carcinoma or urethral stricture. It is also associated with neurological deficits, e.g. diabetes.

If the cause is benign prostatic hypertrophy, *treatments* include alpha-blockers such as doxazosin and tamsulosin, or TURP.

An approach to incontinence

1 Start by asking the patient to keep a voiding diary, recording whether they are continent or incontinent throughout the day, plus chart fluid intake, and any symptoms which might help to diagnose the type of incontinence e.g. incontinence whilst sneezing.

2 Educate the patient about the importance of drinking about 1.5 L of fluid a day, and to reduce caffeine intake as this irritates the bladder.

3 Examine the abdomen for a palpable bladder secondary to obstruction.

4 Rectal examination to assess prostate size in men, exclude faecal impaction and check integrity of anal sphincter.

5 Vaginal examination to exclude senile vaginitis and prolapse.

6 Neurological examination to exclude cord problems.

7 Assess medications: are there alternatives that would not produce large volumes of urine?

8 Education: suggest regular toileting and reduce fluid intake to 1.5 L/day, ensure patient is aware of self-help groups where appropriate.

9 Diagnose and treat any UTIs.

10 Referral to continence advisor.

11 Further investigations such as urodynamics, cystometry and cystoscopy may be indicated if simple interventions fail.

Irreversible incontinence

• Pad and pants are the mainstay.
• The RADAR National key scheme: the Royal Association maintains adapted toilets across the UK for disability and rehabilitation, and they are kept locked. People with disabilities are issued with keys, i.e. RADAR keys.
• Conveens for men, good in theory, but usually fall off too easily.
• Catheters as last resort, to maintain people in their own homes, help carers cope and to protect skin if there is evidence of maceration and to prevent pressure sores.
• Support groups for incontinence such as the National Society for Continence Web site: www.nafc.org.

Vaginal bleeding

Bleeding from the genital tract long after the menopause must always be taken seriously, because there may be pre-malignant or malignant disease as well as benign causes. The patient may present with stained underwear or bed sheets. If she is also incontinent of urine or has an anal lesion, the source of the loss may not be immediately obvious;

however, the history and physical examination should make this clear. The heavier the bleeding, the more likely the cause is to be malignant.

Ask especially about hormone treatment for cancer or hormone-replacement therapy, which is increasingly common; also trauma (including abuse). Even very old women can be subject to this, either from coitus or from some foreign body in the vagina. Further investigation is the province of the gynaecologist. Causes of bleeding are:

• Atrophic vaginitis, which will respond to topical oestrogen cream.
• Benign tumours, such as cervical or endometrial polyps.
• Trophic ulceration from prolapse or foreign body, e.g. ring pessary.
• Endometrial hyperplasia, which may be pre-malignant.
• Cancer of the genital tract, involving vulva, vagina, cervix or endometrium.

Cancer of the prostate

Prostatic cancer is the third most common cause of death in men aged over 55 years. It is very common in the over-70s, when it is usually an indolent condition. However, invasive disease has a mean survival time of 4 years. Screening continues to be highly controversial because, despite much anecdotal evidence of improved outcome in individuals, there is no large-scale research data to demonstrate increased survival rates.

Clinical features

• Often asymptomatic.
• There may be lower urinary-tract symptoms such as poor stream, post-micturition dribbling and nocturia, but usually only late in the disease.
• If the cancer has spread, there may be boney pain or cachexia.
• Rectal examination reveals a hard, craggy prostate.

Investigations

• Measurement of the PSA is readily available, but still lacks sensitivity and specificity.

• The ratio of free to total PSA may give extra specificity. A low ratio implies a greater chance of discovering cancer if the prostate is biopsied.
• Transrectal prostatic biopsy.
• Histology following TURP.
• Bone scintigraphy: a sensitive way of detecting bone metastases.

Treatment

1 Treatment can relieve symptoms but does little to prolong survival.
2 Transurethral resection is necessary to relieve bladder-neck obstruction.
3 If there is evidence of spread beyond the gland, hormone therapy is generally indicated, but not all would agree with treatment in the absence of symptoms, even at this stage. Hormonal 'control' fails eventually, possibly due to 'clonal selection' of hormone-independent malignant cells.
4 Radical prostatectomy gives no better results and the morbidity is greater than with hormonal manipulation.
5 Radiotherapy is also used, especially for the anaplastic tumour (even when still confined to the prostate) and for localized metastases.
6 Occasional blood transfusions are helpful for the patient with slowly progressive metastatic disease and severe anaemia.

In advanced disease, the aim is to reduce androgen stimulation of the tumour to levels found in castrated men, with minimal adverse effects. Loss of libido and potency is inevitable; all current approaches are palliative and include:
1 Bilateral subcapsular orchidectomy is simple, cheap, effective, but can have adverse psychological effects.
2 Antiandrogens, e.g. cyproterone acetate 200–300 mg daily in divided doses, is now a first-line drug despite the extra cost and risk of severe mental depression. More recently, flutamide has been used, with less risk of depression, but with adverse cardiovascular effects similar to stilboestrol.
3 LH releasing-hormone agonists, e.g. goserelin (monthly subcutaneous injections). More expensive than anti-androgens and must be covered by anti-androgen (cyproterone or flutamide) during the first 1–2 weeks of treatment to reduce risk of 'disease flare'.

Sex in old age

Many people continue to enjoy a sexual relationship until the end of life. However, others stop having sex for a variety of reasons:
• Decline in sex drive.
• Erectile dysfunction affects 15–25% of men by the age of 65. It is more common in men suffering from diabetes, hypertension and renal disease, but stress, anxiety and depression play an important part. Premature ejaculation is less common.
• Longer time to arousal.
• Longer time to orgasm.
• Reduced genital sensitivity.
• Loss of lubrication in women secondary to reduced oestrogen.
• Reduced satisfaction.
• Reduced mobility, e.g. from arthritic hips, previous stroke.
• Anxiety about provoking further myocardial or cerebrovascular events. However, the evidence suggests that sex with a familiar partner is unlikely to precipitate a fatal event.
• Disinhibition in one partner secondary to dementia may be off-putting in the other partner.
• Loss of partner, or moving to a residential home with reduced privacy.

Advice for patients to maintain a healthy sex life

• 'Use it or lose it'.
• Plenty of exercise to keep physically fit.
• Do not smoke.
• Avoid excess alcohol.
• Use of artificial lubricants.
• Use of PDE5 inhibitors e.g. sildenafil or tadalafil to achieve erection. [Use contraindicated in patients taking nitrates, or who have history of recent myocardial infarction (MI) or stroke.]
• Consider intermittent catheterization or suprapubic catheter for incontinence.

- Advise that sex does not have to be penetrative, but other physical contact can also be pleasurable.
- Seek help early.

Further information

Brocklehurst, J.C. (ed.) (1984) *Urology in the Elderly*. Churchill Livingstone, Edinburgh.

Dawson, C. and Whitfield, H. (2006) *ABC of Urology*. BMJ Books, London.

Kessel, B. (2001) Sexuality in the older person. *Age and Ageing*, **30**, 121–4.

National Association for Continence. website: www.nafc.org

Royal Association for Disability and Rehabilitation. website: www.radar.org.uk

The National Institute for Clinical Excellence Guidelines on Urinary Incontinence in Women. October 2006. www.nice.org.uk/CG040

Chapter 14

Blood and bone marrow

Introduction

Normal elderly people have normal peripheral-blood films. However, abnormalities increase with increasing age. About one-third of patients will have low haemoglobin. Abnormalities need to be explored and corrected if possible. Haematological changes in old age are important because:

1 They are common.
2 They aggravate other pathologies/symptoms.
3 They are often correctable.

Age changes

The following facts are given because they are interesting, but they are of more theoretical than practical importance.

Red blood cells

There is evidence of reduced deformability in health and this is even more marked in those with cerebrovascular disease.

White blood cells

1 There is more marked granulation (probably due to lysosymes) and lobulation of granulocytes.
2 There is a tendency towards leucopenia, with a normal leucocyte-count range of 3.0–8.5×10^9/L in old age.

3 The lymph nodes, the lymphoid tissue of the GI tract and the spleen are all much reduced. The thymus is atrophied by middle age, but thymic remnants are thought to remain active to extreme old age.
4 The B-cell population is well maintained, but there is a reduction in T-cell numbers and functional capacity.
5 Some impairment of phagocytosis by neutrophils and macrophages has been reported.

Plasma proteins

Conflicting reports on age changes relate to the difficulty in distinguishing those changes due solely to age from those due to other factors, such as malnutrition or disease. The main points to emerge are:
1 Low levels of total protein and of the individual fractions are to be regarded as pathological.
2 Increased globulin fractions indicate disease; however, asymptomatic individuals with very high levels of gamma globulins may have monoclonal gammopathy of unknown significance (MGUS) rather than myeloma.
3 Abnormal immunoglobulins are increasingly common in the very old, present in about 3% of those aged over 70 years and in 20% of those aged over 90.
4 There is an age-related increase in the incidence of autoantibodies and the female preponderance is lost.

Haemopoiesis and ageing

1 There is a gradual loss of active haemopoietic tissue initially in the long bones and later in the flat bones; vertebral marrow persists.

2 The cellular composition of the residual haemopoietic tissue is normal and responds satisfactorily to the usual stimuli, such as erythropoietin, anoxia and blood loss.

Basic investigations

Always request a peripheral-blood film; it is inexpensive and easy and will often lead you directly to the cause and treatment of the blood disease.

Anaemia is the most common abnormality and the red-cell morphology often suggests the aetiology (Figure 14.1). White-cell morphology will also be helpful, especially in myeloproliferative disorders.

Measurement of the acute-phase response is also useful. The ESR is the cheapest investigation but it reflects changes slowly (i.e. days). CRP is better for monitoring more rapid changes (i.e. in hours). Measurement of other plasma proteins by electrophoresis is informative when malignant conditions, such as myeloma, are suspected.

Clinical history and examination

The symptoms of anaemia – tiredness, breathlessness and general malaise – are too common and non-specific to be of great value. Anaemia may exaggerate or exacerbate symptoms due to other pathologies, e.g. angina may become more troublesome, intermittent claudication increases and falls occur more frequently. The patient's symptoms may therefore be greater than expected from the documented haematological abnormality.

The history may help in defining the nature or cause of the anaemia. Ask about dietary change, dyspepsia, change in bowel habit, weight loss, family history (pernicious anaemia), medication and previous surgery, etc.

Physical examination may not be helpful, but it is important to look for jaundice, lymphadenopathy, abdominal organomegaly, rectal masses and neurological abnormalities, as these may direct you to the correct diagnosis.

Investigation of Anaemia

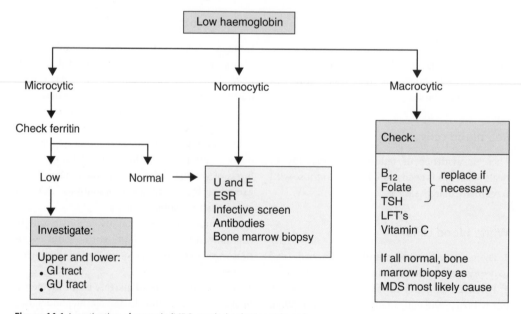

Figure 14.1 Investigation of anaemia (MDS, myelodysplastic syndrome).

Finally, remember that anaemia is a sign of disease and is not a diagnosis.

The types and causes of anaemia

Anaemia is present if the haemoglobin is less than 13 g/dL in males or less than 12 g/dL in females. The main categories are:

1 Red-cell/haemoglobin loss:
 • Due to bleeding.
 • Due to cell destruction (haemolysis).
2 Impaired red-cell/haemoglobin production:
 • Deficiency states.
 • Marrow dysfunction.
 • Anaemia of chronic disease.

Iron-deficiency anaemia (microcytic)

Iron-deficiency anaemia is the most common form of microcytic anaemia: it affects 2–5% of the older population. It is most often caused by bleeding, usually from the GI tract.

Aetiology

1 Iron-deficiency anaemia is usually due to chronic blood loss, especially from the GI tract and, less often, from the genitourinary tract or elsewhere.
2 Defective absorption may be a contributory (rarely the sole) factor. Causes include achlorhydria secondary to chronic gastritis, previous gastrectomy or small-bowel disease. Look for clinical or biochemical evidence of malabsorption, such as steatorrhoea, osteomalacia, folate and vitamin B deficiencies.
3 Inadequate intake may stem from inability to cope as a result of physical or mental disorder or from poverty.

History

1 Symptoms: non-specific, e.g. general malaise, weakness, dizziness, increased number of falls or worsening breathlessness secondary to congestive cardiac failure.
2 Ask about indigestion, change in bowel habit, black tarry stool, weight loss, problems swallowing, blood in the urine, postmenopausal bleeding. The carer may report that the patient is more confused.
3 Restless leg syndrome is sometimes secondary to iron deficiency.
4 Past medical history: gastrectomy, diverticular disease, bowel resections for carcinoma, and so on.
5 Document all drug treatments including over-the-counter medications especially aspirin and ibuprofen.

Examination

See also Chapter 11.
 • General: pallor, lymphadenopathy.
 • Mouth: stomatitis, telangiectasia around the mouth and palate.
 • Hands: koilonychia.
 • Abdomen: epigastric tenderness, masses, scars from previous surgery.
 • Do not forget to examine the rectum for masses and to examine the stool to exclude melaena.

Investigations

 • Peripheral-blood film: the red cells are small and hypochromic. There may also be pencil cells and target cells.
 • Remember that, if there is also B_{12} or folate deficiency, the red cells may not be microcytic.
 • A low serum ferritin is good evidence of iron deficiency. However, it is an acute-phase protein and it may be falsely elevated in the context of infection or inflammation, in which case CRP will be high also.
 • The reticulocyte count can be helpful; if it is raised, this implies bleeding or haemolysis with appropriate increased bone marrow activity.
 • As 10–15% of patients have both upper and lower GI causes of anaemia, most patients need both an oesophago gastro duodenoscopy (OGD) and at least a CT abdomen, progressing to barium enema or colonoscopy where appropriate.
 • OGD will be positive in 30–50% of the cases. All elderly patients should have a small intestinal biopsy to exclude coeliac disease. Upper-GI bleeding is often iatrogenic, e.g. NSAIDs or aspirin.

- Details of investigation and treatment of anaemia secondary to GI disorders are given in Chapter 11.

Treatment

- Iron should be continued for 3 months to replenish the iron stores; it is sufficient to prescribe ferrous sulphate 200 mg twice daily, as more than this may not be absorbed and may cause side-effects such as constipation. Warn the patient that their stools will become black and gritty.
- If the response to oral iron treatment is not satisfactory (i.e. 2 g/dL after 2 months), check that the patient is taking the tablets and that any bleeding has stopped. Also consider additional diagnoses that may explain the problem, such as co-existent anaemia of chronic disease.

Haemolytic anaemia

- A rare form of anaemia in old age and therefore in danger of being overlooked, especially as the peripheral-blood film may not show any specific features, i.e. a variable red-cell size and coloration.
- In this context, these anaemias are usually secondary to immune processes, i.e. as part of an autoimmune illness [e.g. systemic lupus erythematosus (SLE)], due to antibody production secondary to infection (hot and cold antibodies following a viral infection) or as an iatrogenic disease (e.g. the haemolytic anaemia secondary to methyldopa treatment).
- Patients with hypersplenism may also have a haemolytic element to their anaemia.
- Relevant investigations are those indicating increased red-cell destruction, i.e. raised bilirubin level, raised reticulocyte count, haptoglobins and antibody tests (Coombs' test).

Deficiency states causing macrocytosis

The macrocytic anaemias are usually secondary to deficiency of vitamin B_{12}, folic acid or, more rarely, thyroxine. They are much less common than anaemia due to iron deficiency or chronic disease. The bone marrow precursors are megaloblastic, whereas in other causes of macrocytic anaemias (see table 14.1) the bone marrow is normoblastic.

Vitamin B_{12} deficiency

- Pernicious anaemia (PA) is the cause of B_{12} deficiency in 80% of cases in the UK.
- Other causes are gastrectomy, bacterial colonization of intestinal strictures or diverticula and disorders of the terminal ileum, especially Crohn's disease.
- Only strict vegans are likely to suffer from dietary-induced vitamin B_{12} deficiency.

Pernicious anaemia

- Pernicious anaemia develops insidiously due to autoimmune gastric atrophy and failure of intrinsic factor secretion.
- The incidence is said to be 1:10,000 with a female preponderance.
- Cancer of the stomach occurs in about 10% of cases.
- Other complications are peripheral neuropathy, subacute combined degeneration of the spinal cord (i.e. a mixture of corticospinal tract and dorsal column degeneration leading to upper and lower motor neurone signs) and confusion, and these may predate the haematological changes.
- There may be a family history of other autoimmune conditions such as hashimotos thyroiditis, vitiligo, and Addison's disease.

Clinical features

Clinical features include:
- Symptoms and signs of anaemia, with yellow tinge to skin.
- Glossitis, anorexia and weight loss.
- In severe cases, hepatosplenomegaly, heart failure.

Diagnosis

1 The blood film contains large oval red cells and occasionally hypersegmented neutrophils.
2 The bone marrow is megaloblastic.
3 Serum B_{12} is low.
4 The Schilling's (Dicopac double radioisotope) test will confirm that vitamin B_{12} can be absorbed only when given with intrinsic factor. The test is not necessary in most cases.

5 Antibodies to gastric parietal cells are found in the serum in 90%, to intrinsic factor in 60% and to thyroid in 40% of the cases.

Treatment of vitamin B$_{12}$ deficiency
1 Hydroxocobalamin 1mg intramuscularly three times a week for 2 weeks, to replenish body stores and thereafter 1 mg every 3 months for life.
2 There is often associated iron deficiency, necessitating oral iron.
3 Blood transfusion is generally not indicated.

Folate deficiency

Folate deficiency is much more common than vitamin B$_{12}$ deficiency and is usually due to poor diet, with or without malabsorption. Other factors are increased demand, e.g. in lymphoma, neoplasm, infection and haemolysis. Anticonvulsant drugs and chronic alcoholism cause low levels by increasing the hepatic metabolism of folate.

Clinical features
The clinical features include:
1 Irritability, depression, confusion and occasionally dementia.
2 Peripheral neuropathy and subacute combined degeneration of the cord (as with PA) in more severe cases.

Diagnosis
• The peripheral-blood and marrow picture is identical to that of vitamin B$_{12}$ deficiency.
• Red-cell folate is low. Folic-acid absorption tests are not used routinely.

Treatment
1 Correct the aberrant lifestyle – poor diet, alcohol abuse; stop offending drugs, when practicable.
2 Oral folic acid tablets for a few months to replenish stores, and then stop; long-term use may mask developing PA.
3 Do not give folic acid until vitamin B12 deficiency excluded; otherwise there is a risk of precipitating subacute combined degeneration of the cord. If in doubt, give both vitamins concurrently; the patient may need iron also.

4 Prophylactic use in malabsorption states and in epileptics on anticonvulsants may be justified.

Hypothyroidism

The macrocytic normoblastic anaemia, which occurs in over 50% of cases in myxoedema, is usually mild, never megaloblastic and responds slowly to thyroxine. Co-existing iron deficiency will require treatment. About 10% of cases also have PA.

Scurvy

The macrocytic normoblastic anaemia of scurvy is commonly associated with other nutritional deficiencies. Vitamin C is necessary for the reduction of folate into its active metabolite. Vascular purpura occurs and on occasion blood loss can be severe. Vitamin C replacement, followed by a balanced diet, is curative.

Marrow dysfunction

The peripheral red cells are normally normochromic and normocytic but may on occasion be macrocytic. The underlying fault may be inherent in the marrow itself, and examination of the marrow is needed for diagnosis either as an aspirate or a trephine.

Myelodysplastic syndromes

Abnormalities of peripheral-blood film and bone marrow morphology secondary to impaired bone marrow function.
• Incidence increases with age.
• Twenty-five per cent are discovered incidentally on blood film requested for another reason.
• Fifty-five per cent present as a refractory macrocytic anaemia.

Table 14.1 Other causes of macrocytosis.

Alcohol	Myelodysplastic syndromes
Liver disease	Cytotoxic drug treatments
Hypothyroidism	Paraproteinaemia
Reticulocytosis, e.g. due to bleeding/ haemolytic anaemia	Aplastic anaemia

- Twenty per cent present with problems secondary to leucopenia or thrombocytopenia.
- The blood film may show a pancytopenia with giant platelets and juvenile neutrophils.
- The marrow is hypercellular due to stem-cell hyperplasia but poor haemopoiesis.
- A few respond to treatment with pyridoxine, androgens and steroids.
- The majority of cases are best managed with repeated blood transfusions (but remember to consider desferioxamine to prevent iron overload).
- Chemotherapy often too toxic for use in elderly patients.
- Mean survival from diagnosis is 2 years; the illness may end in conversion to a leucaemic picture or the patient may succumb to infections secondary to poor white-cell function.

Aplastic anaemia

- The peripheral-blood picture may be similar to that in the myelodysplastic syndrome but sometimes contains blast cells.
- The marrow aspirate will show depletion in stem cells.
- Most cases are idiopathic.
- Known causes are drugs (NSAIDS, antibiotics, thiazide diuretics and cytotoxic drugs), radiotherapy and toxins (benzene).
- Treatment is supportive with blood and platelet transfusions, and antibiotics for infection. More aggressive therapies include cyclosporin A, antithymocyte globulin, high-dose methyl prednisolone and bone marrow transplantation, but these are best reserved for fit people with no co-morbidities.

Leucoerythroblastic anaemia

An anaemia with immature cells in the peripheral blood. The marrow examination may reveal the malignant cells that have infiltrated and impaired function.

Anaemia of chronic disease

- This is usually a normochromic normocytic anaemia.
- It does not respond to haematinics replacement.
- May be improved by treatment of the underlying condition.
- Seventy-five per cent are associated with malignancy; the remaining cases are associated with infection or inflammation such as rheumatoid arthritis.
- Ferritin is normal or raised.
- There are increased levels of iron in the reticulo-endothelial system.
- The underlying problem seems to be defective iron transfer to red-cell precursors.
- Anaemia of chronic disease can be differentiated from iron deficiency anaemia by measuring the number of transferrin receptors. They are up-regulated in anaemia of chronic disease but normal in iron-deficiency anaemia. This assay is expensive and not yet widely used.

Mixed picture anaemias

Many of these types of anaemia have a mixed picture, with features of deficiencies, blood loss, haemolysis and marrow dysfunction. The blood picture will only improve if the underlying condition can be alleviated. Common examples are as follows.

Rheumatoid arthritis

In addition to 'anaemia of chronic disease', look for blood loss (anti-inflammatory drugs), inadequate nutrition and folate or vitamin B_{12} deficiency. Low folate may be due to reduced intake and increased utilization. Complications of rheumatoid disease, such as vasculitis or amyloidosis, increase the severity and complexity of the anaemia.

Malignant disease

Usually a combination of causes will be operative: anorexia, blood loss, anaemia of chronic disease, malabsorption and haemolysis. Additionally, there may be marrow infiltration, with development of leucoerythroblastic anaemia.

Renal disease

The anaemia in renal disease may be related to the underlying cause, e.g. myeloma or SLE. It is also associated with reduced production of erythropoietin. Elderly patients with chronic renal failure and anaemia are offered subcutaneous recombinant erythropoietin once any iron deficiency is corrected.

Alcohol abuse

Anaemia may be due to a combination of gastric bleeding, duodenal ulceration, dietary deficiency of folate and a direct toxic effect of alcohol on bowel absorption and marrow function.

Myeloproliferative disorders

These malignant conditions are due to uncontrollable proliferation of haemopoietic cells. The predominant cells produced and the speed of progression usually defines the nature of the disease. The diagnosis is usually made on the appearance of the peripheral-blood film and marrow examination.

Acute myeloid leukaemia

Very much an illness of the elderly (over 10/100,000 cases per year in the population aged over 75 years; fewer than 5/100,000 cases per year in all other age groups).

Acute lymphoblastic leukaemia

Mainly a disease of childhood, but highest incidence in adults is in the over-75s.

Treatment of acute leukaemias will combine active chemotherapy and supportive measures. Treatment should only be undertaken in conjunction with a clinical haematologist.

Chronic lymphatic leukaemia

• This is a disease caused by normal lymphocytes living an abnormally long time.

• The aetiology is unknown but there is evidence of a genetic element; it arises at a younger age in successive generations of some families.
• Accounts for 25% of all haematological malignancies.
• Affects older people; the incidence is 50/100,000 per year in the population aged over 70, and this increases with increasing age.
• One-third of cases are detected incidentally on a blood film done, e.g. pre-operative assessment.
• It does not require treatment if asymptomatic.
• May convert to an acute disorder – any intervention should be in conjunction with a haematologist.

Clinical features

• Superficial symmetrical cervical lymphadenopathy.
• Anaemia.
• Hepatosplenomegaly.
• Purpura and bruising secondary to low platelet count.
• Often presents as pruritus.
• Occasionally presents as a florid response to herpes zoster.

Diagnosis

• The blood film contains multiple small lymphocytes and occasional smear cells.
• There may be a normocytic normochromic anaemia.
• Bone marrow aspirate shows replacement of the normal marrow with lymphocytes.

Treatment

Many elderly people have a benign form of the disease, which requires no treatment, and survive for up to 10 years. The mainstay of treatment of those with more aggressive disease is steroids plus alkylating agents. Survival in these cases is usually 3–5 years.

Chronic myeloid leukaemia

Chronic myeloid leukaemia is less common than chronic lymphocytic leukaemia (CLL). It is of

interest because it is the best worked out genetically: the translocation of genes from the long
arm of chromosome 9 to chromosome 22 creating
the Philadelphia chromosome, which produces
an oncoprotein.

- Incidence is 1–1.5/100,000 per year.
- Affects people of all ages, mean range 40–50 years.

Clinical features

- Bone marrow failure.
- Hypermetabolism.
- Splenomegaly may be massive.
- More rarely, leucostasis causing priapism, and
visual impairment; and hyperuricaemia.

Investigations

- Leucocytosis, $50–200\times10^9$/L, with the full spec-
trum of myeloid cells seen in the peripheral-blood
film.
- Bone marrow is hypercellular with granulocytes.
- Philadelphia chromosome may be detected in
the peripheral blood or bone marrow.
- Normochromic normocytic anaemia.
- Platelet count often elevated, but may be normal
or low.
- Raised uric acid.

Progression and treatment

Usually the disease remains in the chronic phase
for 2–3 years. During this phase, it is possible to
treat with chemotherapy and bone marrow transplantation. When the disease enters its acute phase,
deterioration may be rapid, with median survival
being 3–6 months. It is less common than the
lymphatic form but again is found predominantly
in elderly population, and splenomegaly may be
gross. Again, expert haematological guidance is
needed if active treatment is contemplated – usually when conversion to acute form seems
imminent.

Other elements of the blood may also proliferate
to give rise to erythrocytosis and thrombocytosis.
These conditions are rare and their management
requires the expertise of a clinical haematologist.

Myeloma

Myeloma is the abnormal monoclonal proliferation of plasma cells in the bone marrow. It accounts
for 10% of haematological malignancies. It is more
common in men than women and in black populations more than white. It is a disease of older age,
the mean age of onset being 65 years.

The aetiology is unknown, but possibilities include
toxins and the human herpes virus HH8. There may
be a genetic component as it occurs in family clusters.

Clinical syndromes

Common:
- Malaise secondary to anaemia.
- Bone pain and pathological fractures.
- Recurrent infections secondary to immunopare-
sis and neutropenia.
- Renal failure due to deposition of immune
complexes.
- Bleeding secondary to abnormal platelet function.
Less common:
- Confusion secondary to hypercalcaemia.
- Rarely: hyperviscosity syndromes, amyloidosis
or cord compression.

Investigations

- Normochromic normocytic anaemia.
- Red-cell rouleaux.
- Thrombocytopenia.
- Raised ESR and plasma viscosity.
- Hypercalcaemia.
- Abnormal monoclonal plasma-protein band,
usually IgG seen on plasma electrophoresis.
- Bence–Jones proteins (free light chains) in the urine.
- Lytic bone lesions on the skeletal survey.

Treatment

This depends on how the patient presents:
- Careful fluid balance for renal failure, and dialy-
sis in selected cases.
- Fluids and bisphosphonates for hypercalcaemia.
Some studies show that patients treated with
bisphosphonates do better in the long term.

- Radiotherapy for bone pain and cord compression.
- Analgesics, opiates often needed.
- Treat infections, usually bacterial respiratory infections.
- It is important to assess the patient carefully before commencing chemotherapy: consider aggressive treatment with a view to bone marrow transplant in younger and fitter patients.
- If chemotherapy is deemed appropriate, the mainstay is melphalan, usually given with prednisolone. Myeloma usually responds to this but then relapses again.

Monoclonal gammopathy of uncertain significance

Sometimes a paraprotein is found in the serum but there is no definite evidence of myeloma; no bone lesions, no Bence–Jones proteins in the urine.

Some of these patients, but not all, will eventually develop full myeloma.

Lymphoma

There are two main types of lymphoma:

1 *Hodgkin's disease*. This mainly affects adolescents and people in their thirties, but there is a second peak affecting 50–80 year olds. Reed–Sternberg cells are pathognomonic of Hodgkin's disease; they are multi-nucleated giant cells found in the peripheral blood. The clinical features include lymphadenopathy which is typically localized and above the diaphragm. It may be accompanied by constitutional symptoms such as fever and weight loss.

2 *Non-Hodgkin's lymphoma*. The incidence increases with increasing age. Any lymphoid tissue may be affected (up to 20% of cases arise in the GI tract, bone, liver or CNS). Symptoms of both varieties are similar – general malaise, pyrexia of unknown origin, night sweats, pruritus and weight loss. Compression of neighbouring structures may also lead to symptoms. Cerebral lymphoma presents with subacute progression of confusion or other neurological symptoms such as dizziness. It is more common in immunosuppressed patients.

Investigations

- Lymph node biopsy.
- Blood film: leucocytosis.
- Normochromic normocytic anaemia.
- Bone marrow.
- Raised ESR and LDH.
- CT abdomen, pelvis and chest.

Treatment

Treatment depends on histology and staging. The agents used most frequently are cyclophosphamide and chlorambucil, often given with steroids. This is obviously a problem when patients have co-morbidities including diabetes, osteoporosis, heart failure, etc. Thus, each patient must be assessed individually to determine whether or not they would benefit from chemotherapy.

Coagulation disorders

Clotting disorders

- DVT is the most common outcome of a clotting problem in geriatric practice.
- Age alone is a risk factor, but most patients also have other precipitants, such as immobility, trauma (accidental and surgical), underlying malignant disease and dehydration.
- Other conditions in which the blood has increased viscosity, e.g. myeloma, polycythaemia, hyperosmolar non-ketotic diabetic coma and hypothermia, are also complicated by the increased risk of venous thrombosis.
- All patients at increased risk should be offered protection with prophylactic low molecular weight heparin and thromboembolic device stockings (TEDS). See Chapter 9 for more information about venous thromboembolism.

Bleeding disorders

The most common cause of prolonged bleeding is medical treatment or overtreatment with anticoagulants. As the indications for anticoagulation of elderly patients increase, so will the episodes of overtreatment. Elderly patients are particularly at risk, because of the problem of compliance (with both drug regime and regular monitoring) experienced by some elderly patients, plus the complication of drug interactions, especially with analgesics, NSAIDs and antibiotics introduced to treat new problems in patients previously well controlled on regular anticoagulants, not forgetting greater risk of falls, etc.

Other elderly patients at risk are those with thrombocytopenia, whether it is part of their underlying pathology, as in aplastic anaemia or autoimmune idiopathic thrombocytopenia, or as a consequence of powerful chemotherapeutic regimes for myeloproliferative and other neoplastic diseases. The risk of serious haemorrhage, e.g. stroke, is much higher in elderly subjects.

The increasing use of thrombolysis, including streptokinase (see Chapter 9) is another example of elderly patients experiencing both greater benefits and greater risks. Careful selection is needed to avoid the increased risk of bleeding, especially cerebral.

Disseminated intravascular coagulation

In disseminated intravascular coagulation (DIC), thrombosis and bleeding combine. The initial thrombotic element is usually silent but the consumption of coagulation factors used in the process leads to uncontrolled bleeding. The likely precipitants in old age are sepsis, disseminated malignant disease, trauma and fulminant liver failure. Only sepsis is likely to respond to active treatment. Other supportive treatments are blood transfusion for bleeding, fresh-frozen plasma for the replacement of coagulation factors and fresh platelet transfusions. In general, 50% of the patients die, and a higher percentage in very frail elderly patients succumb.

Further information

Bower, M. and Galvani, D.W. (2001) Haematology and oncology. In: *Medical Masterclass* (J.D. Firth, editor-in-chief), Blackwell Science, Oxford.

Provan, D. and Weatherall, D. (2002). *ABC of Clinical Haematology*, 2nd Edn. BMJ books.

Jolobe O.M.P. (2000) Does this elderly patient have iron deficiency anaemia, and what is the cause? *Postgraduate Medical Journal, 76*, 195–8.

Chapter 15

Eyes, ears and skin

Eyes

Age changes

1 Eyes appear sunken in old age due to loss of peri-orbital fat.

2 Arcus senilis is common but not significant.

3 The pupils tend to be small and slow to react to light, and accommodation becomes impaired. Dilatation is also poor and hinders adaptation to dark.

4 Presbyopia is the deterioration of vision with old age. It occurs because the lens becomes inelastic; so that focusing becomes difficult, particularly on near objects.

5 Entropion (in-turned lashes) is common and causes irritation of the cornea. It can be corrected surgically.

6 Ectropion (out-turned lashes) is common and the most frequent cause of epiphora (watery eye). Again, this can be surgically corrected.

Examination of the retinal fundus in old age

Short-acting eye drops are recommended, e.g. tropicamide 0.5%. Reversal with pilocarpine is usually unnecessary and can be painful. The risk of acute closed-angle ('congestive') glaucoma is minimal, but beware the small eyeball with a shallow anterior chamber and small-diameter cornea. If in doubt, dilate only one pupil with phenylephrine 10% and reverse with thymoxamine 0.5% and leave the other eye for a subsequent occasion.

Loss of vision

Approximately 70,000 persons over the age of 65 years in the UK are registered as partially sighted, i.e. about 1% of the elderly population. See Figure 15.1

Causes of Visual impairment

Slow loss:
- Open-angle glaucoma (chronic), 5%: central vision is maintained until late in the disease.
- Cataracts, 33%.
- Age-related macular degeneration, 45%: central vision is lost but peripheral vision is maintained.
- Iatrogenic disease.
- Retinopathy (diabetes mellitus), 17%.

Sudden loss:
- Central retinal artery occlusion, secondary to embolus from carotid bifurcation or mitral valve.
- Venous occlusion: more common in patients with hypertension or hyperviscosity syndromes.
- Retinal detachment.
- Vitreous haemorrhage, more common in diabetics.
- Acute glaucoma.
- Ischaemic optic atrophy, secondary to giant-cell arteritis or atherosclerosis

Note: If one eye is affected, the other is at risk.

Causes of blindness

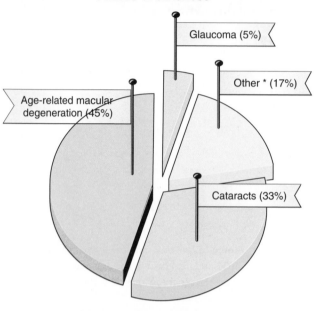

Glaucoma (5%)

Other * (17%)

Age-related macular degeneration (45%)

Cataracts (33%)

* Including diabetic complications

Figure 15.1 Causes of blindness in old age. (*Source*: The Challenges of Aging. ABPI, London, 1991).

Table 15.1 Differences between acute and chronic glaucoma.

	Acute – closed-angle	Chronic – open-angle
Symptoms	Sudden pain in eye, blurred vision, vomiting and prostration	Insidious loss of vision, leading to tunnel vision; family history common
Signs	Eye tense, irregular fixed pupil, cornea and conjunctivae congested	Raised pressure on tonometry, scotoma on field testing; cupped disc
Pathology	Sudden impairment of anterior-chamber drainage – may be precipitated by anticholinergics and mydriatrics	Gradual increase in intraocular pressure – idiopathic
Treatment	Constricted pupil, analgesia, diuretics – urgent action needed	Beta-blockers and/or pilocarpine drops, drainage operation

for the causes of blindness in older people. Many more are visually disabled but remain unregistered. Registration of disability is an essential qualification for special supplementary benefits and aids.

The painful eye

1 Closed-angle glaucoma (acute).
2 Infection:
   (a) Conjunctivitis.
   (b) Uveitis.

(c) Herpes zoster: when the ophthalmic branch of the facial nerve is affected, there may be involvement of the forehead, eyelids and conjunctiva. The patient must see an ophthalmologist urgently.

3 Trauma, e.g. corneal abrasion or a foreign body.

Chronic glaucoma

See Table 15.1 of differences between acute and chronic glaucoma.

- May result in blindness if not treated.
- Early cases best detected by regular eye tests, with ocular-pressure measurement.
- It usually affects peripheral vision first and only affects central vision late in the disease.
- May affect one eye more than the other.
- The intraocular pressure is reduced usually initially with miotic eye drops, such as pilocarpine, or oral carbonic anhydrase inhibitors, such as acetazolamide, or timolol, (a beta-blocker) eye drops.
- If this fails, a trabeculectomy can be performed with an argon laser or surgically.

Acute glaucoma

- Less common than chronic glaucoma.
- Easier to detect because it presents with painful loss of vision.
- The patient may also describe haloes around lights secondary to corneal oedema.
- Treatment is by laser iridectomy.

Age-related macular degeneration

- Tends to affect people aged 50 and over.
- Central vision is affected more, with peripheral vision being preserved.
- Age-related macular degeneration (ARMD) can be divided into two broad types:
    (i) 'Dry' ARMD which tends to develop more slowly and is more indolent.
    (ii) 'Wet' or exudative ARMD, which is more rapidly progressive and causes more visual impairment. Laser treatment has been used with variable results.
- Choroidal neovascularization is an acute change occurring in 'wet' type ARMD caused by new fragile 'leaky' vessels growing into the choroid. This is stimulated by the production of vascular endothelial growth factor (VEGF).
- New treatments have been developed to block the effects of VEGF: pegaptanib sodium (a direct antagonist) and ranibizumab (a monoclonal antibody). Both are given as monthly intraocular injections and probably need to be continued for a least two years to preserve vision. As always, new treatments are very expensive; thus these treatments are likely to create further controversy in the current economic climate.

Cataracts

Very common, easily detected and corrected, resulting in marked enhancement of quality of life.

Types

1 Central – early visual loss.
2 Peripheral – late visual loss and vision impaired by scattering of bright light.

Causes

- Ageing.
- Hereditary.
- Diabetes mellitus.
- Iatrogenic, e.g. steroids.
- Environmental – bright excessive sunshine (the reason for increased incidence in the tropics).

Treatment

Surgery
Timing depends on the needs of the individual, e.g. cataract extraction should be done earlier in those who read a lot, but may be delayed in those whom the distortion and change in magnification and reduced visual fields caused by wearing glasses post-operatively would be a hindrance.

Contraindications
1 Early stages.
2 Where vision is compromised by other ocular co-morbidities such as macular degeneration or severe retinopathy.
3 In the presence of severe mental impairment.

Surgical procedures
- Usually done as a day case under local anaesthetic.
- The anterior chamber of the eye is incised. Phacoemulsification is the process of fragmenting the opacified lens by ultrasound. This debris is removed, leaving the lens capsule intact. An artificial lens is inserted into the capsule.

- Ideally, the power of the new lens is selected to optimize vision so that the patient does not have to wear the thick, old-style aphakic spectacles.

Complications of treatment

1 Dilatation of pupil – may precipitate glaucoma.
2 Lens implant – possible failure and risk of infection.
3 Posterior capsular opacification: may occur several months after the cataract extraction and is treated by Yittrium aluminium Garnet (YAG) laser capsulotomy.

Giant-cell arteritis

See also Chapter 9.
1 This is a vision-threatening disease.
2 Presents with loss of vision associated with headache, usually localized to the temporal arteries plus scalp tenderness when combing the hair, and jaw ache secondary to ischaemia.
3 The patient is often systemically unwell.
4 Examination of the fundus may reveal optic-disc oedema with splinter retinal haemorrhages.
5 The diagnosis is supported by a raised ESR and CRP and confirmed by temporal artery biopsy.
6 The treatment is high-dose oral steroids.

Treatable precipitating/aggravating factors in vascular causes of visual loss

1 Hypertension/hypotension.
2 Diabetes.
3 Polycythaemia.
4 Paraproteinaemia.
5 Arteritis.

Simple measures to assist patients with visual impairment

1 Check visual acuity – provision or change of lenses may help.
2 Keep patient and spectacles together.
3 Keep spectacles clean.
4 Insist on appropriate lighting, a good light is the best visual aid there is. However, some people will benefit from a bright light but glare should be avoided in others.

5 Encourage the patient to be registered as partially sighted or blind. In the UK this is done by a consultant ophthalmologist. The advantages are access to benefits such as attendance allowance, help with telephone costs and cheaper television licences.
6 Seek advice about the availability and use of low-visual aids. Examples include telephones and calculators with large buttons labelled in large print.
7 Maintain maximum hearing ability.
8 Seek support of blind association, e.g. the Royal Institute for the Blind, website: www.rnib.org.uk.
9 Subscribe to talking newspaper, talking-book library, and so on.

Ears

Ageing changes

1 Wax becomes more viscous and needs to be removed in one-quarter of elderly people.
2 Age-related hearing loss (presbyacusis) occurs – loss of high-frequency hearing.
3 Recruitment occurs, i.e. difficulty in hearing when background noise exists.
4 Over 70 years of age, 60% of people have impaired hearing and should be considered for provision of a hearing aid.
5 Impaired hearing leads to impaired health.

Causes of hearing impairment

1 Nerve deafness:
  - Age-related hearing loss (presbyacusis) – the insidious, progressive loss of hearing, most affecting higher pitched sounds.
  - Ototoxicity – drugs, e.g. gentamicin and furosemide in high dosage.
  - Nerve compression, e.g. acoustic neuroma and Paget's disease.
2 Conduction deafness:
  - Impacted wax.
  - Otosclerosis – hereditary condition, therefore early onset likely.
  - Post-infective – chronic suppurative otitis media.
  - Paget's disease of bone.
At present only conductive forms of deafness are amenable to surgical treatment.

Management of hearing impairment

1 Check for wax in ears. This can be removed by first administering softening drops, e.g. olive oil, and then micro-suctioning if necessary.
2 If deafness persists after wax removal – refer for audiometry.
3 If appropriate, a hearing aid should be offered (see the following box).
4 It is worth asking whether or not the patients think they are deaf. If they do not, they are unlikely to comply with a hearing aid.

Hearing aids

• It is important to warn the patient that normal hearing will not be restored by a hearing aid; otherwise, people are so off-put by the noises that they do not persevere.
• Generally, people do better the more they practice with the hearing aid early on.
• For people with bilateral hearing impairment, bilateral hearing aids give the best result, if tolerated.
• Ensure ear mould is inserted correctly into ear; otherwise there will be feedback producing the characteristic whistling noise.
• Teach maintenance of aid, i.e. cleaning of tubing and battery replacement (see Figure 15.2).
• Follow up to ensure that aid is being used – volunteers can help.
• Behind-the-ear analogue hearing aids are the type most frequently used at present.
• Body-worn hearing aids are the strongest available and are therefore still used by people with profound hearing loss.
• In-the-ear aids have the advantage of being discrete but are easily plugged up with wax and are awkward for people with reduced dexterity to fit and they are readily lost, especially in hospitals. They are not useful in patients who have otitis externa (inflammation of the pinna and ear canal).
• The new digital hearing aids have the advantage of being programmed to the individual so that, e.g. the frequency of speech can be amplified and background noise reduced. At present, they are not strong enough for people with severe to profound deafness. They are now available on the NHS.

Note: Digital hearing aids often do not have a volume dial, as the volume is pre-set. Plus they are often switched on just by closing the battery door, which means the batteries tend to run out quickly!

---

5 Inform both the patient and their family about environmental aids, e.g. flashing telephones and doorbells, vibrating-pillow alarm clocks and smoke alarms, and so on. Advise about use of 'T' switch, an aid for use in conjunction with induction loop systems to amplify television, telephones, at cinemas, and so on.
6 Educate the patient about national charities and local support groups.

How to communicate with people who have hearing impairment

1 Do not shout, as this just increases the distortion of your voice.
2 Speak clearly and slowly but not in an exaggerated way.
3 Face the patient and make sure that your face is well lit in order to assist lip-reading.
4 Do not obscure or conceal your mouth; as this makes lip-reading difficult.
5 Ask the patient if they can hear you, adjust tone of voice or try rephrasing your question, and so forth, if problem exists.
6 Check that, if patient has an aid, it is properly worn and functioning.
7 All clinics, consultation rooms and wards should have available a simple portable microphone and earpiece, or 'communicator'.
8 If all else fails, write down your questions.

Complications of deafness

1 Social isolation.
2 Psychiatric disorders, especially paranoia.
3 Associated tinnitus.
4 Associated dizziness and unsteadiness.
5 Increased risk of accidents because of reduced auditory warnings.

Tinnitus

1 Noises in the ears, may be continuous or intermittent. Often described as a rushing, buzzing or roaring in the ears. If full sentences are heard, then a psychiatric cause should be excluded.

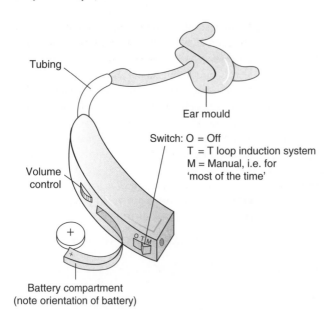

Tubing

Ear mould

Switch: O = Off
T = T loop induction system
M = Manual, i.e. for
'most of the time'

Volume
control

Battery compartment
(note orientation of battery)

Figure 15.2 Behind-the-ear analogue hearing aid.

2 Usually due to degenerative changes in middle or inner ear.

3 If the tinnitus is unilateral, an acoustic neuroma should be excluded.

4 Can be noise induced.

5 Affects over 20% of population over 65 years.

6 Severe symptoms in 5%.

7 Incapacitating in 0.5%.

8 Treatment:
- Hearing aid may help if associated with hearing loss.
- Avoid stress and tiredness as these aggravate the symptoms.
- Try the effect of a masker, which produces 'white noise'.
- Seek support from self-help organization, e.g. Tinnitus Association.

The mouth and its contents

The lips

1 Herpes simplex – as in younger patients, is often an indicator of systemic disease.

2 Angular stomatitis – usually due to escape of saliva due to poor lip closure. The corners of the mouth become red and sore, especially if complicated by fungal (Candida) infection; most common in the edentulous.

Mucous membrane as site of disease

1 Pemphigoid and pemphigus – blisters, see below.

2 Lichen planus – white patches/ulceration, see Table 15.4.

3 Candida – white patches on the tongue or oral mucosa, especially in patients taking oral or inhaled steroids and antibiotics.

4 Aphthous ulcers – as in younger patients.

The tongue

1 Smooth and shiny – iron deficiency.

2 Red and sore – glossitis, e.g. vitamin B group deficiency.

3 Geographical/furred tongue – usually of no significance.

4 Fasciculation – motor-neuron disease.

5 Injury – think of epilepsy.

6 Ulceration – think of malignant disease but trauma from teeth most common cause.

The teeth

1 In the UK 65% of people aged 65–74 years have no natural teeth and this rises to 82% in those over 75 years.

2 In the past, every effort was made to rescue surviving teeth. Modern dentists work to preserve periodontal health as tooth implants are now so effective. It is important to continue having regular dental review; with age the dental pulp atrophies so caries and decay cause less tooth ache than in younger people.

3 Sixty per cent of patients are unhappy with their dentures, usually complaining of looseness.

4 Twelve per cent with dentures never wear them.

5 The edentulous need to continue to consult dentists – gum ridges recede with age and new dentures will be needed.

6 Dentures should only be supplied to those who are prepared to wear them.

7 Dentures should be left in situ in a cardiac arrest, unless they are obstructing the airway.

8 Dignity and nutrition are best maintained if well-fitting dentures are worn by the edentulous; the presence of surviving teeth helps to secure a dental plate and improves the fit.

9 Dentures should be labelled to avoid loss if owner is admitted to an institution.

Note: In wild animals, non-accidental death (i.e. due to 'old age') is most commonly due to starvation secondary to dental loss.

Skin

Age changes

- Confined to the dermis, which becomes thinner, more transparent, more fragile and less elastic.
- The skin in old age is also drier and less greasy, due to reduction in sebaceous excretion.
- There is less subcutaneous fat.
- There is a reduction in epidermal turnover and repair of damage to the skin.
- These two factors reduce the ability of the body to maintain its temperature.
- Reduction in sweating is secondary to both a reduction in the number of sweat glands and in the production by individual glands.
- Reduction in the production of vitamin D.
- Most age changes in the skin are proportional to the extent of environmental damage from sun and wind or heat, as in erythema *ab igne*.
- Age-related blemishes of no significance include senile purpura (on hands and forearms), lentigo on the backs of the hands, Campbell de Morgan spots (on the trunk), sebaceous warts (face and back) and telangiectasia (face).

Damage to skin

Leg ulcers and pressure sores are common, serious and expensive conditions in geriatric practice.

Leg ulcers

These are usually situated in the distal third of the lower leg. When associated with varicose veins, eczema and swollen ankles, they are usually secondary to venous insufficiency. When well demarcated and painful, arterial insufficiency is most likely to be responsible. In many cases there will be a contribution from both venous and arterial disease (Table 15.2).

Treatment

1 Keep clean, warm and hydrated. Cleanse with saline, water or chlorhexidine.

2 Debride wound either surgically or with preparations as per local policy.

3 Cover or pack if large, with paraffin gauze if healing. Use hydrogel, hydrocolloid or alginate dressings if exudate present.

4 Bandage from toes to knee.
- Crêpe bandage in presence of ischaemia or cellulitis.
- Where there is a lot of oedema, four-layer bandaging can help heal ulcers. However, peripheral vascular disease must be excluded (by Doppler measurement if necessary) first.

5 Encourage mobility – but at rest elevate feet.

Table 15.2 Differences between arterial and venous leg ulcers.

	Arterial	Venous
History	Usually recent	Often years
Pain	Present	Often absent
Site	Medial or lateral leg or dorsum of foot	Above medial or lateral malleoli
Appearance	Small, clean, punched out	Large, weepy, infected, surrounding pigmentation or eczema
Pulses	Absent or bruits in proximal vessels (not invariable in diabetes)	Present unless obscured by oedema
Proportion	15%	70%

6 Use antibiotics if there is cellulitis or evidence of sepsis, but avoid topical preparations because of risk of contact dermatitis.

7 Dressings should rarely be changed more frequently than once daily – when healing has started, increase intervals between dressing changes. Hydrocolloid and similar dressings may be left in place for a week.

Cellulitis

This usually presents as painful, red, hot, swelling of the lower limb, and it is often bilateral. If the cellulitis is extensive, the patient may be systemically unwell and have a fever. Care must be taken to exclude a co-existing DVT (see Chapter 5). The most common pathogens are *Streptococcus pyogenes* and *Staphylococcus aureus,* but do not forget MRSA in cases of hospital acquired infection.

Risk factors include chronic leg oedema, trauma causing a pretibial laceration (remember to check whether the patient has been immunized against tetanus toxoid if an injury was sustained in the garden) and maceration between the toes secondary to athlete's foot.

Treatment depends on the severity of the infection. If the patient is unwell, then the best management is admission for intravenous antibiotics, usually benzyl penicillin, adding in flucloxacillin if *Staphylococcus* is suspected. Use erythromycin if the patient is allergic to penicillin. In the case of MRSA, treat with intravenous vancomycin. Oral antibiotics may be used for less severe cases. Treat any co-existing DVT or athlete's foot as appropriate.

Pressure sores

• Areas of necrosis due to persistent and unrelieved pressure that exceeds the perfusion pressure of the tissues.

• Affected areas are usually between bony prominences and an unyielding surface upon which the patient is lying.

• Commonly affected sites include: lower sacrum, hips, heels, shoulder blades, elbows, spine and knees.

• Shearing forces (between the patient's skin and the supporting surface) aggravate the problem.

• Worsened by persistent moisture (e.g. incontinence).

• Expensive: in terms of dressings and increased nursing time.

• Distressing to the patient and their family.

• In debilitated patients, pressure sores may occur within hours, but may take months to heal or even prove to be fatal.

• Prevention is clearly cheaper and more humane than expensive and prolonged treatment.

• However, in many instances the damage may have occurred before presentation, e.g. during a 'long lie' after a fall at home.

• If prevention fails, the extent of the damage must be minimized and healing then encouraged.

• With modern medicine keeping many frail, elderly patients alive and in hospital, the incidence of pressure sores is bound to rise.

• The prevention and management of pressure sores should be multi-disciplinary.

Intrinsic risk factors

1 Poor nutrition.
2 Unconsciousness.
3 Immobility.
4 Cachexia and muscle wasting.
5 Neurological disease.
6 Severe underlying disease.
7 Incontinence.
8 Increased vasoconstriction.
9 Decreased peripheral perfusion.
10 Seventy per cent of all pressure sores occur in the over-70-year-old population.

Extrinsic factors

1 Skin hygiene.
2 Medications, e.g. sedatives, opiates, which would further reduce mobility.
3 Pressure relieving system.

Preventive measures

1 Avoid falls, where possible.
2 Avoid immobility – in bed or chair; delays on hard trolleys in emergency, X-ray departments, and so on, are dangerous.
3 Identify and protect at-risk patients (Waterlow Risk Assessment) (Table 15.3).
4 Relieve pressure when immobility is unavoidable, e.g. by regular turning, mechanical devices (ripple mattress, waterbed, suspension techniques), or protect vulnerable area, e.g. with foam or sheepskin.
5 Monitor the patient's nutrition.
6 Maintain best possible perfusion pressure, i.e. support BP and maintain good hydration.
7 Maintain optimum general health, treat heart failure and maximize haemoglobin level, transfusing the patient if necessary.
8 Keep the skin dry – catheterize if necessary.

Encourage healing

1 Clean the sore, e.g. surgically, by debridement, or chemically, with preparations as directed by local policy.
2 Colloid dressings keep the skin moist and reduce odour, and can often be left *in situ* for several days.
3 Use appropriate systemic antibiotics if there is cellulitis or evidence of septicaemia; include treatment for anaerobic organisms.

4 Give nutritional supplements, including vitamin C and zinc, and correct anaemia.
5 Do not allow deep sores to become sealed off – pack with non-adherent dressings, e.g. colloid or alginate; this encourages healing from the base of the ulcer.
6 If the sore is large, enlisting the help of the plastic surgery team for superficial grafting may be the quickest form of healing.
Do not forget to treat pain.

Pruritus

- This is a common condition in older people.
- It significantly reduces quality of life.
- It can prevent both patient and their carers from sleeping.
- It can cause depression and agitation.
- It is sometimes surprisingly intractable especially in older people who may not be able to apply creams, and so on, on their own because of arthritis, or who are not compliant because of dementia.
- The itch–scratch cycle occurs because scratching causes increased inflammation of the skin and triggers nerve fibres promoting more itch, leading to more scratching and the cycle continues. Eventually the skin is damaged and its barrier function is breeched, allowing superadded infections to occur.
- See Table 15.4 for causes of pruritus.

An approach to management

- Take a good history to make diagnosis where possible.
- Careful examination to exclude infestation/infection or other cause as in Table 15.4.
- Routine blood tests to exclude metabolic cause.
- Keep temperature about 63°F.
- Encourage patient to drink plenty of fluids (at least eight glasses of water per day).
- Avoid hot baths.
- Pat skin dry.
- Moisturize within 5 min of leaving the bath, preferably with a ceramide lipid-based emollient which traps the absorbed water and reduces evaporation.

Table 15.3 Pressure sores: the Waterlow Risk Assessment card.

Build/weight for height	Sex/age	Skin type	Tissue malnutrition	Continence
Average 0	Male 1	Healthy 1	Smoking 0	Complete or catheterized 0
Above average 1	Female 2	Tissue paper 2	Anaemia 1	Occasionally 1
Obese 2	14–49 1	Dry 1	Peripheral vascular disease 1	Catherized and continent 2
Below average 3	50–64 2	Oedematous 2	Cardiac failure 5	Doubly 3
	65–74 3	Clammy 3	Terminal 8	
	75–80 4	Discoloured 4		
	Over 80 5	Broken/spot 5		
Mobility	*Appetite*	*Neurological deficit*	*Major surgery or trauma*	*Medications*
Fully mobile 0	Average 0	Diabetes 0	Orthopaedic below waist 5	Steroids/cytotoxic/anti-inflammatory 4
Restless/fidgety 1	Poor 1	Paraplegia 1	On table for 2 h 5	
Apathetic 2	NG tube/ fluids only 2	MS 2		
Restricted 3	NBM/anoxeric 3	CVA 3		
Inert/in traction 4				
Chair bound 5				

Note: Low risk score - <10

At risk 10–15.

High risk score - 15–20.

Very high risk >20.

NBM: nil by mouth, NG: nasogastric, MS: multiple scleosis.

Table 15.4 Causes of itch in older people.

Cause	Clinical features	Examples	Treatment
Xerosis	Abnormal maturation of keratocytes causes dryness and roughness of skin with fine scale	Associated with PVD and neurological disease	Avoid soap, use emollients
Eczema	Exacerbations in winter/ dry conditions, exposure to allergen	Atopic	Emollients, topical steroids
		Contact	Remove allergen
		Seborrhoeic	Nizorel shampoo to scalp
Psoriasis	Erythematous plaques with silver scale, commonly on extensor surfaces.	Exacerbated by stress, alcohol and drugs such as beta blockers	Treat with topical calcipotriene, Psoralen + UVA treatment (PUVA), methotrexate in severe disease
	Tear-drop lesions on trunk	Guttate psoriasis, triggered by streptococcal infection	
	Lesions on palms and soles	Pustular psoriasis	
Lichen simplex chronicus	Localized raised plaque caused by ha-bitual scratching		Consider covering the lesion with dressing, e.g. Duoderm emollients
Drugs	Ask about new changes in medications	Opiates, phenothiazines, aspirin, quinine,	Stop suspect medications where possible
Urticaria	Type I hypersensitivity reactions to drugs, food, cold, sunlight	Sensitivity to penicillin, sulphonamides, nuts, chocolate	Avoid cause, short course of prednislone
Lichen planus	Itchy purple papules on flexures of wrist	May be triggered by gold and photochemicals	Topical steroids; systemic in severe disease
Dermatitis herpetiformis	Itchy vesicles on extensor sites, buttocks	All patients have gluten enteropathy, but may be sub- clinical	Avoid gluten in diet
Pityriasis rosacea	Itching red rash on trunk in 'Christmas tree' distribution		Usually self-limiting, if necessary try sedative antihistamine or topical steroids
Bullous pemphigoid	Irritating deep bullae		Oral steroids
Infestations	Straight or 's'-shaped burrows in webs of fingers and anterior surface of wrist. Other members of the household will be affected	Scabies	Shower/ bathe in anti-bacterial soap. Topical permethrin solution. Wash clothes and bed-clothes. Treat household and close contacts
Infection	Dermatophytes	Candida in intertriginous areas; Tinea corporis, pedis and cruris	
Neoplasia	Fever, weight loss and itch	Mycosis fungoides Lymphoma	Treat as appropriate
Metabolic	Hypothyroid facies	Hypothyroidism	Levothyroxine
	Uraemic frost	Renal impairment	Relieve cause where possible
	Jaundice	Hepatic impairment	Relieve cause where possible

155

• Educate the patient to avoid scratching: trim fingernails!

• Use steroid creams or ointments for short periods for true inflammatory eczema.

• Consider antihistamines for sedative effect.

• Some people find cooling preparations, containing e.g. menthol, helpful as the coolness masked the itch.

Other important skin conditions in geriatric medicine

1 *Shingles* – the subsequent pain and debility present the most serious aspects of this condition (see Chapter 8).

2 *Pemphigus vulgaris* – this is an autoimmune condition where autoantibodies to the intercellular protein desmoglein Dsg3 cause loss of cell-to-cell adhesion, leading to severe superficial blistering and erosions. The lesions tend to start in the mouth, and then spread to other area of the skin. It is a life-threatening condition because of the high risk of secondary infection and loss of protein. It requires treatment with high doses of steroids. There is much ongoing research into the use of immuno-modulating agents such as tacrolimus and mycophenolate.

3 *Bullous pemphigoid* – a similar but less severe condition. More common in women. The blisters are large and tense because the immunological lesion is deeper in the skin, at the basement membrane. Mouth ulceration is less common. Again, it can be treated with oral steroids, high dose initially until the lesions are under control and then a lower maintenance dose.

4 *Intertrigo* – moist seborrhoeic eczema, which is often secondarily infected with fungi. It is especially common in obese individuals and where there is close skin-to-skin contact under pendulous breasts, abdominal aprons and between the buttocks. Improved personal hygiene and treatment with antifungal preparations will be required.

5 *Solar keratosis, basal-cell carcinoma and melanoma* – especially in fair-skinned people overexposed to sunlight. See squamous carcinoma.

6 *Drug reactions* – can present as any lesion, from eruptions to purpura. Pathological thinning of the skin secondary to steroid treatment is another common example.

7 *Ulceration* – secondary to trauma complicating other pathology.

8 *Rosacea* – typically occurs in older women with fair skins; characterised by erythema, telangiectasia and pustules on nose, cheeks and forehead. Occasionally men develop a severe form with hypertrophy of sebaceous glands and skin of the nose producing the disfiguring rhinophyma. It seems to be triggered by stress, high temperatures, hot drinks and alcohol. Treatment includes oral tetracyclines, topical metronidazol, or topical permethrin. Laser therapy can reduce telangiectasia and rhinophyma.

Malignant diseases of the skin

Predisposing factor in fair-skinned people is excessive exposure to sunlight.

Basal-cell carcinoma

Basal-cell carcinoma (BCC) is the most common skin malignancy. It arises as a pearly papule, usually on the upper face. It slowly, but inexorably, enlarges, and if left untreated it becomes locally invasive. Metastatic spread is rare. BCC is easily removed in early stage by local minor surgery, but larger lesions may require radiotherapy.

Bowen's disease: intraepidermal epithelioma

These lesions appear as single scaly, erythematous plaques, usually in sun-exposed areas. They are squamous-cell carcinomas (SCCs) that have not invaded beyond the epidermis. They are treated with cryotherapy, surgical excision or radiotherapy.

Squamous-cell carcinoma

Squamous cell carcinoma is less common than BCC. It presents as a reddened, indurated ulcer, nodule or plaque. SCC often arises in sun-exposed areas, e.g. in a solar keratosis or patch of Bowen's disease, but also in other situations where the skin has been damaged such as in chronic venous ulcers. It may metastasise to lymph glands. Once the diagnosis is confirmed by biopsy, it should be excised or treated with radiotherapy.

Malignant melanoma

These are expanding pigmented lesions, again usually, but not always, arising in sun-exposed skin. They require early excision because of risk of metastases.

Hair and nails

Age changes

1 *Hair* – becomes thinner and more brittle and loses its natural colour. Baldness may occur in both sexes but with differing distribution. Body hair is lost in the same order as its acquisition. Facial hair increases in women.
2 *Nails* – become thicker and harder – onychogryphosis when extreme.

Pathological changes

1 Retention of hair colour is said to indicate hypothyroidism. If the hair is extra dry, this also may be a sign of hypothyroidism.
2 Exaggerated hair loss may indicate hypopituitarism or Addison's disease, or be a consequence of cytotoxic therapy.
3 Toe nails may be neglected because of difficulty with maintenance due to visual impairment, arthritis or stroke disease.

4 Brittle and deformed nails may indicate systemic disease, e.g. deficiencies such as calcium or iron. Clubbing, pitting and white bands may indicate disease elsewhere.
5 Discomfort due to toe nail deformity and neglect can seriously impair mobility.
6 Extra care is needed in nail maintenance in patients with peripheral vascular disease and neuropathy, especially diabetics.

Further information

Baum, B.J. (1992) *Clinics in Geriatric Medicine – Oral and Dental Problems in the Elderly*. W.B. Saunders, Philadelphia, PA.
Fook, L. and Morgan, R. (2000) Hearing Impairment in older people: a review. *Postgraduate Medical Journal*, **76**, 537–41.
Finlay, A.Y. (ed.) (2000) *Dermatology Parts 1 & 2*. *Medicine*, Vol. 28: 11 and 12, The Medicine Publishing Group Ltd.
Gilchrest, B.A. (ed.) (1989) *Clinics in Geriatric Medicine – Geriatric Dermatology*. W.B. Saunders, Philadelphia, PA.
Royal National Institute for the Blind Web site: www.rnib.org.uk
Macular Degeneration website: www.macula.org
Royal National Institute for the Deaf website: www.rnid.org.uk
Willot, J.F. (1991) *Ageing and the Auditory System*. Whurr Publishers, London.
NICE Guidelines for the pressure ulcer prevention (www.nice.org.uk/CG029).

Chapter 16

Legal and ethical aspects of medical care of elderly people

Introduction

Most elderly patients pose no more ethical or legal problems than other adults. However, in a few, particularly where there is mental as well as physical frailty, problems are numerous. Some of these issues have recently been dragged into the spotlight, with accusations of 'ageism' and 'medical paternalism' being hurled at anyone who dares to suggest that it is sometimes in a patient's best interest to be a little economical with the truth or less than heroic in efforts at resuscitation. Some of the legal aspects are straightforward, others less so. Ethical problems are often resistant to dogmatic resolution.

Driving in later life

The *law* of the land obliges everyone to surrender their driving licence at the age of 70. A new licence is then issued, which is valid for 3 years but can be renewed every 3 years on completion of a declaration of good health. The *insurance company* may insist on a medical examination. The Driver & Vehicle Licensing Authority (DVLA) must be advised of any change in health status. Certain conditions will render the individual unfit to drive:

• Episodic impairment of consciousness (e.g. epilepsy, hypotension, severe vertigo, poorly controlled diabetes).
• Paroxysmal symptomatic cardiac arrhythmia and severe ischaemic heart disease (e.g. angina at the wheel).

• Severe Parkinson's disease.
• Fluctuating or declining cognitive function.
• Uncorrectable visual impairment, particularly significant field defects.
• MI, pacemaker insertion, stroke with good recovery or transient ischaemic attack – for at least a month.
• Always check details of the length of driving restrictions on the DVLA website. Advice for elderly drivers includes:
• Avoid distractions such as chatty passengers and changing CDs.
• If a long journey is unavoidable, take adequate breaks.
• If the route is unfamiliar, make advance preparations and allow plenty of time.
• Avoid peak traffic times and night driving.

Ethical difficulties may arise in this connection and two are common:

1 The patient refuses to accept advice to stop driving despite one of the disorders listed earlier.

2 The patient may have a degree of cognitive impairment but, even though they do not have one of the proscribed conditions, the doctor is convinced they are unsafe.

3 If you are advising someone to stop driving, present it in terms of 'the other drivers on the road – so much more traffic, drivers are less courteous these days, I am worried that if someone else did something silly e.g. mother let a child run out, that it might take a little longer for you to weigh up

the options', etc. If the doctor is unable to persuade them to give up driving, a family member may be prepared to try to do so, particularly if they have firsthand experience of a terrifying ride in the passenger seat. Suggest seeking the opinion of a professional driving instructor or a session at a driving assessment centre. However, if a patient continues to drive after advice to stop, then it becomes the doctor's duty to the public to inform the DVLA (make the patient aware of your intention).

The Mental Capacity Act (MCA) 2005

This comes into force in 2007 and is a statutory framework:
• To empower and protect vulnerable adults who are not able to make their own decisions ranging from the daily, e.g. what to eat, to the occasional but serious, e.g. consent to surgery.
• To enable people to plan for a time when they may lack capacity.

Who needs to know about the MCA?

If you have a patient who lacks capacity, this may affect how they are managed in a number of ways:
1 If they are to be discharged from hospital to different accommodation.
2 If decisions are to be made about serious medical treatment, e.g.:
  • Decisions about surgery.
  • Medical investigation.
  • Cancer treatment.
  • Renal dialysis.
  • Feeding tubes.
3 If they are to be included in drug trials.
  The MCA will affect how you consult family and friends and the patient may need an advocate.

Serious medical treatment

This is defined as providing, withdrawing or withholding treatment where:
• For a treatment there is a fine balance between benefits/burdens and risks e.g. deciding whether or not to amputate a gangrenous foot in a patient who has just had a stroke.

• Choice of treatments is finely balanced e.g. type of chemotherapy in advanced breast cancer.
• What is proposed would have serious consequences for the patient.

Five principles that MCA underpinned

• There is presumption of capacity, unless demonstrated otherwise.
• Individuals should be supported to make their own decisions.
• People retain the right to make an eccentric or unwise decision.
• Others must act in the best interests of the patient.
• If an intervention is needed, it should be the least restrictive.

Assessment of capacity

This is only considered if the patient has impairment of brain function. Capacity is decision- and time-specific, i.e. a person may be able to decide what to eat and to make a will, but may not be able to decide about returning home. However, the situation may be different tomorrow.

In order to have capacity, the person must be able to:
1 *Understand* the information relevant to the decision (consequences of deciding one way or another or failing to make the decision).
2 *Retain* that information for long enough to decide (even though they may then forget a decision had been made).
3 *Use* that information as part of the process of making the decision.
4 *Communicate* the decision (any method including sign language, squeezing the hand, etc.).

Advance decisions

Currently, 'advance directives' have force under common law. The MCA will put the status of their successor, advance decisions on a statutory footing. A person:
1 Can specify what treatment they would not want and under what circumstances.
2 Cannot demand treatment.

To be valid, the advance decision must have been made when the person had capacity. It is only applicable to the circumstance described, e.g. 'I do not want resuscitation if I cannot speak after a stroke' will not influence treatment after a heart attack. To refuse life-sustaining treatment, the advance decision must be in writing, signed and witnessed and specify 'even if life is at risk'. If the person is detained under the Mental Health Act (MHA), this takes precedence.

Lasting Power of Attorney

This is the method by which a person with capacity can choose who will look after his affairs in the future if capacity is lost.
1 Replaces Enduring Power of Attorney, which only looked after property and affairs.
2 The donor confers on the *attorney* (a person of their choice, usually a relative or friend, not a lawyer) authority to make decisions about all or any of:
 • Donor's health and personal welfare.
 • Donor's property and affairs.
3 Lasting Power of Attorney (LPA) must be registered (Office of the Public Guardian)
4 If your patient lacks capacity and has a personal welfare LPA, the attorney will discuss the patient's treatment with you.

A patient who has a moderate estate but does not have capacity to take out a LPA should have their affairs placed in the hands of the Court of Protection. Application may be made by a relative, the solicitor or the doctor. A medical certificate is required and the court will usually appoint an interested relative or other suitable person as a deputy, to act as the patient's agent, but not to dispose of assets. Where the assets only consist of social security benefits, the Department of Social Security can nominate an *appointee* to deploy them for the person's benefit.

Court of Protection

This is a new specialist court that:
1 Declares whether or not a person has capacity, if there is dispute.
2 Make decisions about health care/treatment.

3 Make decisions about property/financial affairs.
4 Appoint deputies (previously receivers) to have ongoing authority.
5 Make decisions in relation to LPA (and their predecessors' enduring powers of attorney).

The court can issue a declaration that a proposed treatment would be lawful. In considering the patient's best interests, the court will be guided by the *Bolam test,* which simply asks whether the treatment would be supported by a responsible body of medical opinion. An approach to the court is best made through the hospital's legal services manager or, in an emergency, through the duty manager. One source of uncertainty is whether a refusal to be treated reflects a depressive illness and it may be necessary to seek a psychiatric opinion. People are allowed to make unusual decisions: the judgement in the highly publicized case of 'Miss B' in the UK in 2002 gives a strong steer to the profession that, providing the patient is competent, the stated wishes should be respected however apparently irrational. The public guardian and his office run the affairs of the court. It is now a criminal offence to mistreat a person lacking capacity.

Independent Mental Capacity Advocates (IMCA)

1 Most people who lack capacity have support from family and friends (or an attorney or deputy).
2 If there is no such person (or they are 'not practicable or appropriate' to consult) and a decision is needed about serious medical treatment (not emergency) and change of accommodation, there is a duty to instruct an IMCA. They will need access to and be able to copy health/social care records.
The duties of an IMCA:
1 Support the person who lacks capacity and represent their views and interests to the decision maker.
2 Obtain and evaluate information.
3 Ascertain the person's wishes, feelings, beliefs and values.
4 Ascertain alternative courses of action.
5 Obtain a further medical opinion if necessary.
6 Challenge a decision if necessary in the patient's interests.

Consent

Consent must be sought for all medical interventions, although this will often be a very informal process and sometimes only implied. Without it, the health care professional has committed the crime of *battery*. Written forms are highly desirable for surgical procedures and research involving drug trials or other interventions, although oral consent is equally valid in law. Consent must be *informed*, which means that the doctor must provide the necessary information, and ambiguities can arise concerning just how much information has been imparted and whether it was couched in appropriate and readily assimilable terms. Consent must also be voluntary; in other words, no undue pressure must have been exerted on the patient.

Emergency symptomatic treatment of the incompetent patient

In practice, this implies the parenteral sedation of the acutely confused, disturbed patient whose restlessness or aggressive behaviour is a danger to himself or herself or, less commonly, to others. It is permissible under common law to hold the patient down to administer an injection in these circumstances as a last resort and for his or her own protection, if other physicians would regard it as appropriate and if reasonable people would want the treatment themselves. The procedure is deeply distressing to one and all and can usually be avoided (see also Chapter 4).

Restraints

Sedation is a form of chemical restraint and has been termed a 'pharmacological straitjacket' but may be temporarily necessary in the acutely confused, ambulant patient until investigations and treatment rectify the condition. Patients seldom fall out of bed: they fall while trying to get out of bed; so fitting bedrails ensures that the fall occurs from a greater height than it otherwise would, and nursing them on a very low bed or even a mattress on the floor may be preferable. Lethargic but frail subjects may receive some protection from bedrails, which remind them to ask for help to go to the toilet and thereby prevent them from slithering from the side of the bed to the floor. Tilting or 'bucket' chairs should be avoided where possible, but poor staffing levels and a rising tide of complaints and litigation has made the prevention of falls by any means a higher priority for management than respect for autonomy.

Environmental restraints

Environmental restraints include doors that, although not locked, are difficult to open, or a barricaded kitchen in the home, both occasionally necessary for the individual's protection. The gas supply to the cooker may be disconnected and hot meals may be delivered. A controversial restraint is the *electronic tag*, which triggers an alarm if the patient leaves the hospital ward. This may infringe civil liberties but less so, perhaps, than having your life support systems switched off as you lie in ITU by a disorientated patient who wanders in and wants to plug a toaster into an inconveniently occupied socket. Whatever type of restraint is used, the method, the reasons and the arrangements for review should be documented.

Testamentary capacity

Testamentary capacity means mental competence in the single connection of drawing up (or revoking) a will. In order to be capable of this act, a person needs to:
• Understand the nature of such an act.
• Have a reasonable grasp of the extent of their assets – so an assessing doctor has to have at least a vague idea of the patient's circumstances.
• Be aware which persons have some claim on their property.
• Be free of delusions which might distort their judgement.

The Mental Health Act (1983)

Section 2 – admission for assessment

• Applicant – nearest relative or approved social workers.

- Signatories – two doctors – one must know the patient (preferably the GP), the other having special experience.
- Duration – 28 days.

Section 3 – admission for treatment

- Signatories – as above.
- Duration – up to 6 months, unless consultant discharges patient sooner.

Section 4 – emergency admission

- Applicant – as above – must have seen patient within past 24 h.
- Signatory – any doctor.
- Duration – 72 h.

Section 5 – holding power

Allows forcible detention of informal patients being treated for physical or psychiatric problems, for up to 6 h by a qualified mental illness nurse if doctor unavailable: consultant or deputy may enforce the detention for 72 h.

Section 7 – guardianship

On grounds of mental disorder and in the interests of the patient's welfare, a guardian may be appointed who can cause the patient to reside in a given place, attend for treatment (but not necessarily take it) and allow access to a doctor or approved social worker.

- Applicant – as above.
- Signatories – two registered practitioners.
- Guardian – local authority social services or any other person.
- Duration – up to 6 months.

Guardianship is more widespread in Canada and the US than in the UK.

The government signalled its intention to reform the MHA in a white paper in 2000, but there has been ongoing controversy and the latest version is still being debated (2007). The main changes are likely to include:

1 Introducing supervised treatment in the community.

2 Broadening the range of professionals who can take on key roles in the MHA.

3 Improving patient safeguards by creating a set maximum period before which patients must be referred to the tribunal which reviews their detention but improving public safeguards by removing finite restriction orders.

4 Introducing a simplified single definition of mental disorder, so that patients do not fall between the four current categories.

5 Introducing a new requirement that appropriate treatment must be available if patients are to be subject to detention for treatment or supervised community treatment.

National Assistance Act (1948, amended 1951)

Section 47 – removal to place of safety

This is used extremely rarely as a last resort to remove a frail old person from a situation of self-neglect that appears life-threatening or endangers others and the person refuses to cooperate. The GP, social worker or police may apply to the director of public health for compulsory removal to a geriatric or psychogeriatric ward or a residential care home. The authority of a magistrate is required and the duration is 3 weeks. The section is intended to enforce removal when it is likely that this will substantially improve the patient's health. Specialist advice is needed in view of recent human rights legislation.

Ethical issues relating to life-supporting interventions

Cardio-pulmonary resuscitation

Cardio-pulmonary resuscitation (CPR) is the issue that ferments the most emotion. This is because of massive publicity in the media, which has led to a widespread misconception by the public that the 'do not attempt resuscitation' (DNAR) decision by hospital staff is the major determinant of life or death during the admission. There is a great deal of pressure on staff to introduce this topic at their first encounter with the patient. Yes, it is important, but it does not apply to death from any disease except cardio-respiratory arrest, and it does not often work outside the coronary care unit (CCU): about 20% of patients survive CPR, but only about 14% will leave hospital, and only 4% of those will be over the age of 75. It is a procedure about which patients, relatives and hospital staff harbour unrealistic expectations.

A DNAR decision should be taken by the most senior doctor available, after discussion with the patient, if applicable, the team, and with the permission of the competent patient, the relatives, regularly reviewed, and recorded in the notes, together with the reason, under the following circumstances:

• Where CPR is not in accordance with the sustained wishes of the patient.
• Where successful CPR would be followed by a quantity and quality of life that would be unacceptable to the patient.
• Where the patient already has a poor quality of life that he or she does not wish to have prolonged.
• Where effective CPR is unlikely to be successful – e.g. the treatment is futile. This would apply to patients with:

1 Advanced terminal cancer (death expected in days or weeks).
2 Sepsis.
3 Pneumonia on admission.
4 Renal failure.
5 Hypotension.
6 Severe disability.
7 Deteriorating consciousness, e.g. severe stroke.
8 Arrest due to GI haemorrhage.

However competent the patient, no discussion needs to be held in this situation.

A recent statement on the subject of CPR carries authoritative guidance. It should be clearly understood that a DNAR decision is not a proxy for other decisions and does not imply 'not for treatment' – the patient will continue to receive appropriate treatment for their condition.

The intensive care unit

The usual reason for considering a request for an ITU bed is to access respiratory support, e.g. by ventilation, for life-threatening respiratory failure due to airway obstruction, pneumonia, neurological disorders or drug overdose. The dilemma is to avoid deaths when the cause is reversible (asthma, Guillain–Barré syndrome) but also the prolongation of life when the outlook is hopeless (end-stage emphysema, motor-neuron disease). The other considerations are similar to those governing CPR – the patient's and the relatives' wishes and the previous quality of life. Unlike cardiac arrest, one of the commonest causes of respiratory failure, COPD, is predictable, and will end in respiratory failure; so the patient's wishes can, ideally, be ascertained while they are well. Age *per se* is not a bar to ventilation.

Invasive methods of nutrition and hydration

The British Medical Association (BMA), supported legally by the historic Bland case, considers that the use of nasogastric (NG) tubes and percutaneous endoscopic gastrostomy (PEG) tubes, and, by analogy, intravenous fluid administration, constitute medical treatment. If unlikely to benefit the patient, there is therefore no obligation to provide it. Where it is not benefiting the patient, it is permissible to discontinue it, although it may be necessary to seek the court's approval, especially in cases of persistent vegetative state (PVS). As in other forms of treatment, the patient's wishes are the key issue – with incompetent patients, their wishes if known and, if not, their best interests with input from the family, friends or an IMCA.

No method of feeding is risk-free. Even oral feeding and drinking, which constitute basic care rather than treatment, may lead to choking and aspiration. NG tubes are often associated with reflux and aspiration, and PEGs with skin infections and tube blockage – nor do they prevent aspiration. Thirst in the aspirating patient can be relieved by mouth care. Stroke victims and those with terminal cancer often pose emotive ethical dilemmas in relation to giving or withholding fluids and nutrients. In the former case, except where the prognosis looks hopeless, it should initially be assumed that good recovery is possible and nutrition provided by 72 h after the event in those still unable to feed by mouth. For those who feel very uncomfortable with a visibly dehydrating terminal patient, it has been stated that 'the ethical situation is not that the patient is failing to drink and therefore will die, but that the patient is dying and therefore does not wish to drink'.

Age discrimination

Ageism is another hot topic, and is said to remain widespread throughout the UK's NHS, despite the measures outlined in the government's National Service Framework for Older People. In a book on geriatric medicine, the easy option would be to make a sweeping condemnation of it as an evil similar to racial or gender discrimination. When based upon blind prejudice, this may be so. But age discrimination is often based on three rational and humane, if misconceived, principles:

• Older people are denied access to high-tech interventions on the basis that they do much less well than younger ones. There are usually studies available that indicate just how beneficial each intervention is for elderly subjects; to use chronological age as a proxy for cardio-respiratory, functional and cognitive assessment is lazy.

• The potential quantity and quality of life are too low to justify the procedure under consideration. Life expectancies for the otherwise well elderly are surprisingly high, even at advanced ages and the quality of life of an old person can only be assessed by that person and is consistently underestimated by doctors and others.

• To make such interventions available to older patients is to deny them to younger ones. It is not the role of physicians to compare how deserving their patients are. Politicians should not flinch from accepting the responsibility for rationing when resources are inadequate.

Elder abuse

Old age abuse is difficult both to define and to detect. It takes many forms:

• Physical – pushing, punching, slapping, overdosing or withholding medication.
• Psychological – verbal abuse, shouting, swearing, blaming, humiliating.
• Financial – 'asset-stripping'.
• Emotional.
• Neglect – withholding food, drink and warmth.
• Sexual.
• Cultural – e.g. forcing a vegetarian to eat meat.
• Studies in the UK and the USA suggest a prevalence of such abuse in 5–10% of the dependent older people.

Risk factors

Victim
• Heavy dependency, communication difficulties
• Behavioural problems, aggression

Shared
• Poor housing
• Poor long-term relationship

Carer
• Excessive alcohol consumption
• Changed lifestyle due to caring role
• Divided loyalties, e.g. elderly parent and child
• Health problems, including psychiatric
• Role reversal – ageing child and aged parent
• Isolation, real or perceived

Detection

Although the diagnosis is difficult to substantiate, there are some warning signs:

• Recurrent falls and accidents, unexplained fractures.
• Multiple bruising, especially clear thumbprint bruises to arms sustained while being shaken, or bruises or burns to unusual areas such as flexure surfaces.
• Injury similar in shape to an object.
• Patient tries to hide a part of the body from examination.

• Patient withdrawn, frightened (especially of carer), anxious, makes effort to please.
• Carer complaining of 'nerves' or of being under stress.
• Difficulty gaining access to patient.
• Isolation of patient in one room of home or care setting.
• Refusal by patient and/or carer to accept necessary support services.

Action to be taken

A competent older person has the right to choose to remain in a vulnerable setting and, if they wish to do so, may be very reluctant to admit to what is going on. Any discussion must be held in private and, if there are grounds for suspicion, the matter must be pursued through interdisciplinary channels, as there should be a local lead professional or agency.

Euthanasia

If euthanasia is taken in its literal sense of 'a good death', we must all be in favour of it, although most are opposed to the practice of the more generally accepted definitions:
• *Voluntary euthanasia:* the deliberate and intentional hastening of death at the request of a seriously ill patient.
• *Involuntary euthanasia:* ending a person's life without seeking their opinion.
• *Non-voluntary euthanasia:* ending a person's life for their benefit, when they cannot possess or express views whether they should live or die.
• *Physician-assisted suicide:* the patient takes a lethal cocktail by himself or herself that has been prescribed or provided by the physician at the patient's request.

All of these forms of *active euthanasia* remain illegal in the UK, although it is perfectly acceptable morally and legally to administer increasing doses of sedative and analgesic drugs that may, incidentally, shorten life (which they actually seldom do), if the doctor's intention is to provide effective pain relief – the so-called 'double effect'.

To withhold potentially life-prolonging treatment is sometimes called *passive euthanasia* and some ethicists regard it as morally indistinguishable from active euthanasia. But, as we have seen, no doctor is obliged to initiate or continue treatment that they consider futile.

Breaking the bad news

There is little evidence as to whether there are right ways to do this unpleasant duty, although there are certainly wrong ones. There are a few generally accepted guidelines:
• A trusted and familiar doctor or nurse (better still, both) should, ideally, do it in the presence of a close family member (unless the patient raises an objection).
• Ensure privacy, identify the relatives and introduce yourself.
• Pre-plan the discussion and sit down to indicate that you have plenty of time. Avoid jargon; do not be afraid of eye contact, physical contact or silence.
• Try not to kill all hope or to give a precise forecast of the duration of the illness. Offer a second opinion, if wanted.
• Do not be afraid to speak of death and dying but avoid forcing the issue and only give as much information as they can cope with, undertaking to meet again.
• Do not strive for too much detachment – patients and relatives often appreciate it if they see that the doctor or nurse is affected emotionally.
• Undertake to continue support and to relieve symptoms.
• Record what was said, and to whom, in the notes.

There is a danger that, in insisting on observing the patient's right to know, we may neglect the patient's right *not* to know. It is usually sensible to take *some* notice of a relative's plea. 'For Heaven's sake don't tell him – it would kill him', but not to be bound by it. But we have all met many patients who make it clear that they do not wish to be burdened with diagnostic and prognostic information, and firmly answer, 'No, I don't think so, thank you' when we enquire if they have any questions they would like to ask. It is only humane to continue to offer the opportunity but not to force the issue.

There is also the danger that we break the rules of confidentiality by informing relatives without the explicit consent of a competent patient. The team of carers is different, because they are all bound by a similar ethical code, but this may not apply to the manager of a care setting and it is something we should constantly bear in mind.

Death certification

After a death at home, the doctor should see the body to confirm and certify death. In hospital, deaths are commonly confirmed by the nursing staff. The certificate is then completed by the hospital doctor, except in those cases where the coroner needs to be informed.

Her Majesty's Coroner

Doctors must exercise their judgement in individual cases, but when in doubt, ring the coroner's office. The following deaths should normally be reported:

• Death of a person not attended by a doctor during their last illness.

• Death of a person not seen by a doctor either within 14 days before death or after death.

• When the cause of death is unknown.

• Deaths after accidents including falls, misadventure, starvation, severe deprivation (neglect) including hypothermia, poisoning.

• Drugs, whether therapeutic or of addiction, or abuse, including alcohol.

• Anaesthetic, surgical or medical mishap or when relatives express serious dissatisfaction or allege neglect.

• Deaths within 24 h of emergency admission (unless the GP is happy to sign the death certificate) or within 24 h of an operation.

• Industrial diseases, even if not a cause of death.

• Septicaemia of possible unnatural cause.

• Those with disability pensions from service with the Crown.

• Prisoners and anyone in the custody of the police.

Further information

Action on elder abuse: http://www.elderabuse.org.uk/

BMA ethics advice: http://www.bma.org.uk/ap.nsf/Content/Hubethics

Driving: http://www.dvla.gov.uk/media/pdf/medical/aagvl:pdf

GMC advice on withholding and withdrawing life-prolonging treatments, including artificial nutrition and hydration and CPR: http://www.gmc-uk.org/guidance/current/library/witholding_lifeprolonging_guidance.asp#78.

Mental Capacity Act:

Office of Public Sector Information: www.opsi.gov.uk/acts/acts2005/20050009.htm

Department of Constitutional Affairs: www.dca.gov.uk/legal-policy/mental-capacity/publications.htm

Department of Health: http://www.dh.gov.uk type IMCA into search. Redley report.

Example of an agency proving IMCAs in Cambridge: http://www.speakingup.org/

Mental Health Act: http://www.mind.org.uk/Information/Factsheets/ and type in Mental Health Act.

National Assistance Act: http://www.healthprotection.org.uk/ and type in National Assistance Act.

Chapter 17

Palliative care

Age, place and cause of death

Almost 80% of the deaths in the UK occur in people aged 65 and above, and almost 65% of women die aged 75 or over. Sadly, perhaps, the majority of all deaths occur in institutions, as Table 17.1 shows.

Ischaemic heart disease, cancer, stroke and respiratory failure are the leading causes of death in the UK and most other developed countries. Of these, terminal cancer and end-stage cardiac, respiratory and renal failure are the conditions that alert the clinician to the inevitability of a fatal outcome, and enable the team to switch the emphasis of treatment from cure to the relief of suffering and the preservation of dignity. Ethical and legal aspects of 'end-of-life decisions' are considered in Chapter 16.

Table 17.1 Place of death.

Percentage of deaths	Location
54	NHS hospitals
13	Private hospitals, nursing homes and residential care homes
4	Hospices
29	Own home or elsewhere (e.g. public places)

Symptom control

Pain

It is important to try to analyse the source of the pain, as certain types of pain require rather specific measures to relieve them. Examples include:

1 *Neuropathic pain*, in which tricyclic antidepressants, anticonvulsants, such as gabapentin or valproate, ketamine, or transcutaneous electrical nerve stimulation (TENS) are more likely to be successful than conventional analgesics. Nerve blocks and other specialist interventions may be required.

2 *Bony metastases*. NSAIDs or intravenous bisphosphonates are often helpful. Hormonal treatment usually relieves the pain of prostatic secondaries, and a single bony deposit will respond well to radiotherapy.

3 *Headache due to raised intracranial pressure*. Dexamethasone 16 mg a day is given for a week and then reduced by 2 mg a week to a level of 4–6 mg daily. Remember to give it in the mornings as it raises levels of alertness.

4 *Nerve compression*. Dexamethasone 8 mg orally a day is often helpful, but local infiltration may need to be considered.

5 *Stretching of liver capsule by metastases*. Prednisolone up to 25 mg a day can be helpful.

6 *Intestinal colic due to bowel obstruction*. Antispasmodics can be used such as hyoscine hydrobromide 0.6–2 mg by subcutaneous infusion. Octreotide

reduces intestinal secretions and therefore can reduce symptoms. It is given subcutaneously 300–600 mcg over 24 h.

Pain in general falls into the two categories of acute and chronic. The acute type of pain lasts for 2–4 h and analgesia can be given when required in standard doses. Chronic pain, however, requires analgesics to be given in anticipation of the pain and with the aim of a long duration of action. The dose will require titration for the individual patient at that particular stage of his or her illness. In the context of terminal palliative care, it is the latter type of pain that is most frequently encountered. The principles are the same whether the pain is due to malignant disease or to other causes, such as an ischaemic limb, which is not amenable to reperfusion surgery and which the patient is unwilling to have amputated. The usual concept is that of the 'analgesic ladder'. This implies a long and weary climb to the top, whereas in practice the number of steps is usually only two or three:

1 *Paracetamol*, given regularly has been proven to reduce even severe pain.

2 *Failing this, it is usual to use a synthetic opioid analogue*. Meptazinol is a useful partial opioid agonist, and tramadol is relatively free from adverse effects.

3 *Strong analgesics*, which are usually used in a regular dosage regime, often with the addition of less strong analgesics between doses for 'topping-up' purposes for 'breakthrough' pain. In the UK, the principal preparations are morphine and diamorphine, although the latter is illegal in other countries, notably the US, where hydromorphone is extensively used instead. Diamorphine is claimed to cause less nausea than morphine, and is certainly more soluble, permitting the injection of smaller volumes. In addition to their analgesic properties, these drugs have a valuable euphoriant effect and induce a pleasant state of detachment.

The main problems associated with the use of morphine and diamorphine are as follows:

1 *Drowsiness*, which many patients find highly unacceptable. They can, however, be assured that it usually wears off within a few days.

2 *Constipation* is universal. A strong laxative such as co-danthramer, which combines lubricant and stimulant properties, should routinely be prescribed.

3 *Nausea*. This can usually be overcome by the use of antiemetics (see Table 17.2), but usually wears off in any case.

4 *Respiratory depression, cough suppression, hypotension* – seldom limits use of these agents.

5 *Tolerance and addiction*. The former is easily overcome by increasing the dose and the latter can be disregarded as irrelevant.

6 Oral, rectal or transdermal use is to be preferred to *repeated injections*, but if the latter are necessary, e.g. due to intractable vomiting, diamorphine is preferable because of its greater solubility and the smaller volumes therefore required. A syringe driver is extremely useful in this situation, with a subcutaneous needle, usually using the anterior chest wall, with the addition of an antiemetic if necessary.

A practical guide to the use of opiates in palliative care is given in the box below.

Opiate usage

1 Start with oral morphine sulphate solution or tablets 5 mg regularly 4 hourly (if a double dose is given last thing, it should last through the night). Oramorph® solution contains 10 mg/5 mL and there is a concentrated solution containing 20 mg/mL.

2 Increase dose until pain relief is adequate.

3 Convert to morphine sulphate modified-release tablets, capsules or suspension: total dose in 24 h is identical but given in two equal doses. The MXL preparation has a 24-h duration. A non-opiate or comparable 'rescue' doses of immediate-release morphine can be given for 'breakthrough' pain.

4 To convert to morphine injections, use half the oral dose of morphine. To convert to diamorphine injections, use one-third the oral morphine dose (the same applies to intravenous morphine). Usual route is subcutaneous, by syringe driver if needed regularly.

5 Fast acting fentanyl 'lolly pops' provide a boost of analgesia to cover pain from dressing changes and so on.

6 Fentanyl and buprenorphine transdermal patches provide analgesia for 72 h. Conversion tables from oral morphine are available. They have the advantage of allowing free mobility.

Table 17.2 Causes and treatment of nausea and vomiting.

Clinical features	Clinical pattern	Causes	Drug Treatment
Persistent, severe nausea; little vomiting	Chemical/ metabolic	Uraemia Hypercalcaemia Chemotherapy Opioids, opiates	Haloperidol Granisetron
Intermittent, mild nausea; large volume vomiting; early satiety	Gastric stasis/ outflow obstruction	Drugs including opioids, anticholinergic Local tumour Hepatomegaly	Metoclopramide
Dysphagia with little nausea. Nausea relieved by vomiting	Regurgitation	Oesophageal or mediastinal disease	Dexamethasone
Intermittent nausea, improved by vomiting. Vomiting large volumes which may be faeculent, sometimes with little warning. May be associated pain, abdominal distension, constipation	Bowel Obstruction	Malignant; tumour in lumen, within bowel wall or pressing on bowel wall. Benign: post op adhesions, secondary to radiotherapy Faecal impaction, constipating drugs, oedema of bowel wall secondary to inflammation	Metoclopramide if no colic, Hyoscine butylbromide if colic present. Octreotide Cyclizine and or haloperidol Granisetron
Headaches, nausea, worse in the mornings	Cranial disease	Cranial tumour Cranial radiotherapy Raised intracranial pressure	Cyclizine dexamethasone
Mixture of above symptoms	Unclear/ multiple causes	Combination of above causes	Levomepromazine

Anxiety and depression

Minor tranquillizers or antidepressants are used as required, and antidepressants can also potentiate the effect of analgesics. Psychostimulants (dexamphetamine or methylphenidate) have been found useful in some cases of depression.

Restlessness and confusion

Physical causes should be sought, such as a distended bladder or rectum or a respiratory or urinary-tract infection. If restlessness and agitation persist, a major tranquillizer will be required. Haloperidol 5 mg intramuscularly is often successful and this can be followed by 5–10 mg daily in divided doses.

Nausea and vomiting

It is important to identify the cause: see Table 17.2 for antiemetics.

Anorexia and malaise related to hepatic metastases

Prednisolone 20 mg a day is often extremely successful for these unpleasant symptoms.

Breathlessness

The cause should be identified and appropriate treatment given. The following types of dyspnoea require specific management:

1 *Superior vena cava obstruction*. This is an oncological emergency and should be treated by radiotherapy. Dexamethasone 16 mg a day can be used meanwhile, if there is any delay.

2 *Lymphangitis carcinomatosa*. Dexamethasone is sometimes of value.

3 The *'death-rattle'* due to sections inadequately cleared by dying patients. By this stage, the patient is generally clouded, but it is the relatives who experience considerable distress as a result of this phenomenon. Hyoscine hydrobromide at a dose of 400 µg 4–8 hourly is injected with the purpose of drying up the secretions.

4 *Pleural effusions*. Occasionally these do not reaccumulate following drainage, but most often they do. It may be necessary to call upon the respiratory physicians to attempt pleurodesis, using, e.g. intrapleural tetracycline.

Other common causes of dyspnoea, such as bronchospasm, cardiac failure, pulmonary emboli or anaemia, are treated along conventional lines.

Multiple pulmonary metastases, radiation fibrosis and other causes of dyspnoea should be treated using opiates or diazepam and/or oxygen, whichever gives the best symptomatic relief. Ongoing work suggests that a battery-operated handheld fan can reduce the claustrophobic fear caused by breathlessness.

Offensive fungating tumours

Radiotherapy is often helpful. The local application of metronidazole ointment should also be considered.

Bowel obstruction

Surgical intervention is clearly inappropriate where there is extensive carcinomatosis, as indicated by liver metastases on ultrasound examination or significant ascites. The 'drip and suck' regime should be avoided where possible in this situation and the pain can be best relieved by continuous subcutaneous diamorphine infusion. Colicky pain should be alleviated by means of subcutaneous hyoscine butylbromide (Buscopan®) 60 mg or so in 24 h. As vomiting is likely to be a problem, strong parenteral antiemetics and octreotide may well be required. A phosphate enema or laxatives can be used to try to relieve the associated constipation, and patients who respond to these measures can be permitted small quantities of food and fluid.

Other problems and some solutions

• *Hiccough*: use metoclopramide or chlorpromazine.
• *Dysphagia*: consider stent or laser treatment for oesophageal carcinoma.

- *Dry or painful mouth* (poor oral hygiene or thrush): good mouth care, artificial saliva such as Biotene Oral Balance; treat thrush with fluconazole.
- *Diarrhoea*: treat cause.
- *Constipation*: treat cause, prescribe laxative if using opioids.
- *Cough*: oxygen, opioids, local anaesthetic lozenges, hyoscine.
- *Insomnia*: try to analyse cause.
- *Hypercalcaemia*: treat if symptomatic.
- *Ascites*: drain if causing discomfort.
- *Spinal-cord compression*: radiotherapy if diagnosed early.
- *Lymphoedema*: pressure device, support.
- *Pruritus*: attention to hygiene, use of emollients instead of soap.

Syringe Drivers

When the patient is so unwell that they are unable to take any medications orally, but are distressed, using a subcutaneous syringe driver is an excellent method of providing symptom control.

- Diamorphine for pain and severe agitation/distress.
- Remember to co-prescribe an antiemetic: consider cyclizine, haloperidol or methotrimiprazine.
- Midazolam is useful to terminate fits and also sedate terminally restless patients.
- Hyoscine can also be added to the pump to reduce respiratory secretions.

The Liverpool Integrated Care Pathway for the Dying Patient

- Aims to enable all patients to have a dignified death.
- It supports the family and others, by making it clear that the patient is dying and that the focus of care is now symptom relief. It enables ward staff to explain that some symptoms such as the 'death rattle' are more distressing to the relatives than to the patients
- It provides pre-emptive prescribing for symptom relief so that the patient does not have to wait for treatment.

- It helps to address patients' spiritual and religious needs.
- Provides educational support to patients, relatives and the medical and nursing staff.

Enabling people to die at home

In the majority of cases, it is possible to control symptoms adequately by means of the foregoing measures. The pain service and the palliative care nurses offer specialist expertise in difficult cases.

In 90% of cases in which dying patients are admitted to hospital (or to a local nursing home provided that the diagnosis has been established and a care plan prepared) the reason is the inadequacy of community support – either because the relatives are unduly stressed or because of unavailability of adequate nursing. Where the community nursing service is unable to meet the increasing care needs of the terminal cancer patient, Marie Curie nurses can augment the amount of support available and advice on symptom control from Macmillan nurses will help to support the primary-care team. Where there is a local hospice, its outreach team can again supplement the care available in the community and may even offer short-term admission for the purpose of achieving symptom control where this has proved difficult in the patient's own home. Practical advice and support are often available through patient support groups.

Bereavement

After the age of 75, 30% of men and 64% of women are widowed. Four main phases of grief have been described, but the stages vary enormously with each individual and few people progress steadily through each stage in a logical way.

1 Shock and disbelief. This is characterized by numbness, disbelief and an inability to accept what has happened.

2 Yearning. This phase may be characterized by acute pangs of severe loss and pining and a restless searching for the dead person, who often appears in dreams and hallucinations. Periods of guilt and anger

are directed at oneself or the dead person or other family members and friends and hospital staff.

3 Depression and apathy. This is a time of hopeless despair, with periods of joyless monotony. It is often associated with profound depression and loss of self-confidence, and guilt and anger are again common features. This emotional turbulence may continue for a year or more.

4 Acceptance. This involves the acceptance of the reality that the loved person is dead and that life has changed, and the bereaved person resumes a lifestyle that, to a greater or lesser extent, has become adapted to his or her new status. This phase enables the bereaved person to let go of the dead loved one and to start a new sort of life.

The first of these phases may last for days and the second for weeks. The third phase is likely to last for a number of months, but most people adjust to a major bereavement within 1–2 years. Hallucinations, in which the dead person is vividly seen, may continue for a prolonged period. However, mourning is associated with a number of tasks, which include acceptance of the reality, experiencing the pain, adjusting to the new environment and redirecting energy towards new relationships and activities. An inability to work through the phases of grief is sometimes called a pathological grief reaction and is particularly likely to occur following sudden or untimely deaths. There is a high incidence of ill health and death in the surviving spouse following bereavement. Most areas of the UK now have a branch of the charity CRUSE, which exists to offer help of many different kinds to bereaved people where it is needed.

Further information

Billings, J.A. (2000) Recent advances: palliative care. *British Medical Journal*, **321**, 555–8.

British National Formulary (Current Edition). Chapter on Palliative Care. BMJ Publishing Group Ltd.

Liverpool Care Pathway for the Dying Patient: http://www.lcp-mariecurie.org.uk/.

Twycross, R.G. (1999) *Introducing Palliative Care*, 3rd Edn. Radcliffe Medical Press, Abingdon, Oxfordshire.

Cruse Bereavement Care Website: www.cruse bereavementcare. org.uk/

Appendix 1

Standards for long-term care

Patients in long-term care, in both the public and independent sectors, are amongst the most vulnerable to abuse and neglect. The following checklists and audit systems are recommended.

Patient-orientated facilities and services
- Are there separate toilets for men and women?
- Are patients taught new skills?
- Can patients go to bed when they wish?
- Is there a notice board?
- Are there smoking and non-smoking areas?
- Does each patient have a lockable cupboard?
- Is there a patients' committee?

Privacy
- Is it available when required?
- Is it available for telephone calls?
- Is it available for visiting sessions?

Architectural choice
- Is there a shop?
- Are there both showers and baths?
- Are there chiropody and hairdressing rooms?
- Is there a 'television-free' lounge?

Personal amenities
- Does each patient have an accessible bedside light?
- Does each patient have an accessible electric socket?

Socio-recreational
- Is there a garden accessible to patients?
- Are there views from the windows?
- Is there a visitors' room?

Engagement
- Are patients encouraged to maintain skills?
- Is self-help encouraged?
- Do patients and staff sit and talk together?

Further reading

Age Concern advice on choosing a care home: http://www.ageconcern.org.uk/AgeConcern/fs29.asp

Commission for social care inspection: http://www.csci.org.uk/

Counsel and Care fact sheet on what to look for in a care home:

Fahey, T., Montgomery, A.A., Barnes, J. and Protheroe, J. (2003) Quality of care for elderly residents in nursing homes and elderly people living at home: controlled observational study. British Medical Journal, 15(326), 580. Full free text: http://www.bmj.com/cgi/content/full/326/7389/580

Institutional elder abuse (2006) *Lancet,* **367**, 624.

The Barthel Scale

Feeding	2 = independent: reasonable speed
	1 = needs help; e.g. cutting, spreading butter
	0 = unable
Bathing	1 = independent
	0 = dependent
Grooming	1 = face/hair/teeth/shaves all alone
	0 = dependent
Dressing	2 = independent; ties shoes; copes with zips, etc.
	1 = needs help, but does half in reasonable time
	0 = dependent
Bowels	2 = no accidents
	1 = occasional accidents/needs help with enemas, etc.
	0 = incontinent
Bladder	2 = no accidents; manages catheter alone, if used
	1 = occasional accidents, or needs help with catheter
	0 = incontinent
Toilet	2 = independent
	1 = needs help
	0 = unable
Bed/chair transfer	3 = totally independent
	2 = minimal help needed – verbal/physical
	1 = able to sit, but needs major help
	0 = unable – lifted bodily
Ambulation	3 = independent for 50 m – may use aid
	2 = 50 m but with help of person – verbal/physical
	1 = wheelchair but independent – 50 m
	0 = immobile
Stairs	2 = independent
	1 = needs help – verbal/physical
	0 = unable
Total	
	(Max. score = 20)

Appendix 3

CAGE questionnaire for alcohol problems

The CAGE questionnaire is a short screening instrument commonly used in the clinical setting, especially primary care. Ask your patient:

> **C** Have you ever felt you should cut down on your drinking?
> **A** Have people annoyed you by criticizing your drinking?
> **G** Have you ever felt bad or guilty about your drinking?
> **E** Eye opener: Have you ever had a drink first thing in the morning to steady your nerves or to get rid of a hangover?

The CAGE can identify alcohol problems over the lifetime. Two positive responses are considered a positive test and indicate further assessment is warranted.

Further information

Ewing, J.A. (1984) Detecting alcoholism: The CAGE questionnaire. *Journal of the American Medical Association*, **252**, 1905–7.

The Abbreviated Mental Test (AMT)

Each question scores one mark

1	Age
2	Time (to nearest hour)
3	Address for recall at end (e.g. 42 West Street)
4	What year is it?
5	Name of institution
6	Recognition of two persons
7	Date of birth (day and month)
8	Year of First World War
9	Name of present monarch
10	Count backwards from 20 to 1
Total	(out of 10)

Source: Hodkinson, H.M. (1972) Evaluation of a mental test score for assessment of mental impairment in the elderly. *Age and Ageing*, **1**, 233–8.

A score of 7 or below is likely to indicate impaired cognition (but indicates the need for further assessment as the person could be delirious, demented, depressed, deaf, non-English speaking or just not impressed with your questions). The test is also criticized for requiring knowledge of British history, but it is still widely used.

The Geriatric Depression Score (GDS)

Depression is common in the elderly. The 15-point Geriatric Depression Score (GDS) is a useful screening tool

1	Are you basically satisfied with your life?	**No**	Yes
2	Have you dropped many of your activities and interests?	**Yes**	No
3	Do you feel that your life is empty?	**Yes**	No
4	Do you often get bored?	**Yes**	No
5	Are you in good spirits most of the time?	**No**	Yes
6	Are you afraid that something bad is going to happen to you?	**Yes**	No
7	Do you feel happy most of the time?	**No**	Yes
8	Do you often feel helpless?	**Yes**	No
9	Do you prefer to stay at home, rather than going out and doing new things?	**Yes**	No
10	Do you feel you have more problems with memory than most?	**Yes**	No
11	Do you think it is wonderful to be alive?	**No**	Yes
12	Do you feel pretty worthless the way you are now?	**Yes**	No
13	Do you feel full of energy?	**No**	Yes
14	Do you feel that your situation is hopeless?	**Yes**	No
15	Do you think that most people are better off than you are?	**Yes**	No

Score one point: **No** to **1, 5, 7, 11, 13**: **Yes** to **2, 3, 4, 6, 8, 9, 10, 12, 14, 15**

A score indicating depression includes positive and negative answers but, unless you are very stressed, you will be able to work this out! A patient scoring 0–4 is not depressed, a patient scoring 5–15 requires further assessment

Appendix 6

Fitness to fly

1 The partial pressure of oxygen falls at high altitude, even in pressurized aircraft. The resulting 3% reduction in saturation of arterial blood can be significant to patients with severe cardio-respiratory disease and those with a haemoglobin level of less than 8.8 g/dL. Supplementary oxygen during flight will compensate.

2 Dehydration may occur because of the reduced humidity at high altitude – fluid intake must therefore be maintained.

3 Extra space may be required by passengers with disabilities: this may be particularly important on economy flights.

4 Patients with mobility problems may not be able to cope (unassisted) with the arrangement of space at airports.

5 Post-operative patients, up to 10 days after abdominal or chest surgery, may run into difficulties because of gas expansion (e.g. in gut or pleural space) at high altitudes.

6 Colostomies may function more frequently than usual during a flight.

7 Epileptic attacks become more likely.

8 Confusion may be precipitated in vulnerable patients by reduced oxygen levels dehydration anxiety and 'jet lag'.

9 Immobility and dehydration may precipitate DVT.

Advice to passengers

• Always advise the airline of medical problems so that special arrangements can be made, e.g. extra oxygen, extra space, mobility aids and special diets.

• The cabin crew is not trained in nursing – special staff may need to be employed.

• Airlines retain the right to refuse to transport passengers they consider unsuitable.

Respiratory function in the elderly

Appendix 8.1 FEV1 and FVC (mean values) in the elderly.

Age (years)	Sex	FEV1	FVC
62–70	Male	2.18	3.17
	Female	1.63	2.02
70–79	Male	1.92	2.85
	Female	1.43	1.80
80+	Male	1.97	2.89
	Female	1.01	1.45

Note: FEV1, forced expiratory volume in 1s; FVC, forced vital capacity.
In the original, values are given for different heights.
Source: Milne, J.S. and Williamson, J. (1972) Respiratory function tests in older people. *Clinical Science*, **42**, 371–81.

Appendix 8.2 Peak Expiratory Flow Rate (L/Min) in the elderly (predicted values).

Age (years)	1.50 m (4′11″)	1.55 m (5′1″)	1.60 m (5′3″)	1.65 m (5′5″)	1.70 m (5′7″)	1.75 m (5′9″)	1.80 m (5′11″)
65	443	468	483	498	513	528	543
	311	330	349	367	386	405	424
70	435	449	464	478	493	507	522
	301	320	338	357	376	394	413
75	423	438	452	466	480	494	508
	290	309	328	346	365	384	403
80	412	426	440	453	467	481	495
	280	299	317	336	355	373	392
85	410	414	428	441	454	468	481
	269	288	307	325	344	363	382

Note: Upper figures are for males and lower for females.
Source: Cotes, J.E. (1979) *Lung Function*, 4th Edn. Blackwell Scientific Publications, Oxford.

Malnutrition Universal Screening Tool (MUST)

Step 1 BMI score	+	Step 2 Weight loss score	+	Step 3 Acute disease effect score

BMI kg/m^2 Score > 20 (> 30 Obese) = 0 18.5–20 = 1 < 18.5 = 2	Unplanned weight loss in past 3–6 months % Score < 5 = 0 5–10 = 1 > 10 = 2	If patient is acutely ill and there has been, or is likely to be, no nutritional intake for > 5 days score 2

Step 4
Overall risk of malnutrition

Add scores together to calculate overall risk of malnutrition
Score 0: low risk, Score 1: medium risk, Score 2 or more: high risk

Step 5
Management guidelines

0 Low risk	1 Medium risk	2 High risk
Routine clinical care Repeat screening Hospital–weekly Care homes–monthly Community–annually For special groups, e.g. those > 75 years	*Observe* Document dietary intake for 3 days if subject in hospital or care home If improved or adequate intake–little clinical concern; if no improvement–clinical concern–follow local policy Repeat screening Hospital–weekly Care homes–at least monthly Community–at least every 2–3 months	*Treat* * Refer to dietitian, nutritional support team or implement local policy Improve and increase overall nutritional intake Monitor and review care plan Hospital–weekly Care homes–monthly Community–monthly * Unless detrimental or not benefit is expected from nutritional support,. eg. imminent death.

All risk categories:	*Obesity:*
Treat underlying condition and provide help and advice on food choices, eating and drinking when necessary. Record malnutrition risk category. Record need for special diets and follow local policy.	Record presence of obesity. For those with underlying conditions, these are generally controlled before the treatment of obesity.

Index